Antioxidants
Your Complete Guide

D0150222

How to Order:
Single copies may be ordered from Prima Publishing, P.O. Box 1260BK, Rocklin, CA 95677; telephone (916) 632-4400. Quantity discounts are also available. On your letterhead, include information concerning the intended use of the books and the number of books you wish to purchase.

Antioxidants
Your Complete Guide

Fight Cancer and Heart Disease, Improve Your Memory, and Slow the Aging Process

Carolyn Reuben

Prima Publishing
P.O. Box 1260BK
Rocklin, CA 95677

© 1995 by Carolyn Reuben

All rights reserved. No part of this book may be reproduced or transmitted in any form or by any means, electronic or mechanical, including photocopying, recording, or by any information storage or retrieval system, without written permission from Prima Publishing, except for the inclusion of quotations in a review.

Production by Steven Martin
Interior design and layout by Marian Hartsough Associates
Copyediting by Mike Rutherford
Cover design by The Dunlavey Studios

Library of Congress Cataloging-in-Publication Data

Reuben, Carolyn, 1947-
    Antioxidants : your complete guide / Carolyn Reuben.
    p. cm.
    ISBN 1-55958-522-6 (pbk.)
    1. Antioxidants—Health aspects. 2. Free radicals (Chemistry)—Pathophysiology. 3. Vitamins in human nutrition. 4. Medicine, Preventive. I. Title.
    RB170.R48 1994613—dc20
    [347.306482]
                                               93-49709
                                                 CIP

94 95 96 97 98 RRD 10 9 8 7 6 5 4 3 2 1
Printed in the United States of America

This book is dedicated to the one for whom I've
    waited a lifetime,
the prince who made the fairy tale come true,
the "rock" who's been a loving Abba for Natanya,
a soul mate for me,
the only one to whom I said "forever,"
the one and only Allen.

Contents

Part II   Preventing and Healing Disease with Antioxidants   77

Part III Gathering Further Information 205

Acknowledgments

For their kindness in taking time out of extremely busy schedules to critique chapters and share their expertise, I thank the following researchers, writers, and inspired deliverers of light: Jeffrey Blumberg, Ph.D. (Antioxidants Research Lab, Tufts University); George E. Bunce, Ph.D. (Virginia Polytechnic Institute); Robert F. Cathcart III, M.D. (Los Altos, California); Richard Hammerschlag, Ph.D. (City of Hope, Duarte, California); Barbara Marinacci (Linus Pauling Institute, Palo Alto, California); Aleksandra Niedzwiecki, Ph.D. (Linus Pauling Institute, Palo Alto, California); Robert Rowan, M.D. (Anchorage, Alaska); Arline Salbe, Ph.D. (Department of Medicine, Cornell University Medical College); Elena Servinova, Ph.D. (Department of Molecular and Cell Biology, University of California, Berkeley); Raymond J. Shamberger, Ph.D. (Omegatech King James Medical Laboratory, Cleveland, Ohio); Roy L. Walford, M.D., Ph.D. (Department of Pathology, University of California, Los Angeles); Richard Weindruch, Ph.D. (Department of Medicine, University of Wisconsin); John H. Weisburger, Ph.D. (American Health Foundation, Valhalla, New York).

For their part in making the book a reality, I thank senior editor Jennifer Basye Sander for choosing me, project editor Andi Reese Brady for setting the creative course, Mike Rutherford for editing with a good-humored and professional hand, and project editor Steven Martin for shepherding this book efficiently and sensitively to completion.

For creating medical research materials of incalculable worth, I thank authors Melvyn R. Werbach, M.D., and Kirk Hamilton, PA-C.

For allowing me to follow my brother, Rabbi Steven Carr Reuben, through the publishing door at Prima, I thank Prima's founder and president, Ben Dominitz.

For walking ahead in so many admirable ways, as a book author, speaker, and general expert in the fine art of living a meaningful life, I thank brother Steven.

For the fine illustrations, I thank Lisa Zdybel, an excellent artist and a warmly generous neighbor.

For coming into my life when I desperately needed research assistants, I thank Maury Silverman in Washington, D.C., and Murray Fins and Irene Arredondo in Sacramento.

For her friendly reception and assistance, I thank Dorothy Thurmond, librarian (Guttman Library, Sacramento–El Dorado Medical Society).

For serving as my agent, I thank Barbara Lowenstein and her able staff, particularly Robert Ward and Norman Kurz.

For believing in me, supporting me in every possible way, serving as models of self-care, and instead of saying I'm too far out saying I'm ahead of the crowd, I thank my parents, Betty and Jack Reuben.

For letting me know that family matters, no matter what, I thank my remarkably able sisters, Ronna Mallios and Debra Reuben (who have books in them, too, yet to be written).

For cleaning, cooking, chauffeuring, cheering, and keeping the new family humming until "PB" (post-book), I thank Allen Green.

For patiently waiting until the book was done so you could "get on with your life," I thank my precious and precocious daughter, Natanya.

And thank you, dear reader, for your kind attention to what follows. Without you, all the efforts of everyone else I've mentioned would be for naught. May you find the information useful.

Author's Note

What follows is the result of many months of collecting information from the world medical journals, from researchers who read my first drafts, and from phone interviews with physicians who use nutrition in their daily medical practice. Please do not confuse information with medical advice.

When using nutrition for healing, the same rules apply as when taking a drug. Dosages differ from one person to another. Each person's biochemistry is unique, and that uniqueness can make one person suffer miserable headaches after a few weeks of 20,000 IU daily doses of vitamin A while another feels great taking 50,000 IU.

Neither I nor the publisher knows your unique needs. Find a good nutritional guide through the resources listed in Part III, or read widely and deeply to educate yourself. And, before you dive into the pool of self-care, ask yourself if you are willing to take on the responsibility and risk that go with it.

If you have any questions or comments, I welcome your correspondence through the publisher's address printed on the title page. Thanks!

Introduction

The best bakers don't use rancid oil. The best carpenters don't use rotted wood. When the best results are desired, each profession uses the best raw materials possible. We don't often think of ourselves as an end result, yet we too are the product of a variety of raw materials, including what we put into our mouths. Although for thousands of years alert physicians have noticed a direct connection between food and health, it is only within the past couple of decades that scientists have figured out why this is so.

It appears that oxygen, our old friend, is also an intimate enemy. Why should this element of nature be any different from other aspects of life on earth? Fire warms and disfigures; water slakes and suffocates. The same plants that are poisons are also medicines. In all cases, what is valuable at one dose and form is dangerous in another.

The villain in this unfolding story isn't oxygen as we know it in the fullness of our lungs. As described in "The High Cost of Free Radicals" (Part I), scientists are blaming fragments of the gas, with names like singlet oxygen, superoxide, hydroxyl, and peroxides, for cancer, heart disease, cataracts, rheumatoid arthritis, the skin and organ changes associated with aging, and other health problems.

At first you may want to ignore the issue entirely as one more danger described in the morning's news. However, this news is different. This time the headlines are focused not only on the cause of your misery but also on the easy availability of your cure. As easy as opening the refrigerator. As easy as breakfast, lunch, and dinner. Not one meal or two, but years of breakfasts, lunches, and dinners of the right sort.

What is the right food to improve health? Do you really need nutritional supplements? What are the "antioxidants" that are now so widely advertised? These are the questions this book answers.

In Part I you'll meet wayward free radicals, which some believe are the roots of disease and aging. You'll find out what makes an oxidant bad and an antioxidant good. Next appear The Four Aces, a special group of antioxidant nutrients that act as minute superheroes to save the day, and your life. These four superheroes have several herbal and nutritional pals that help them do the job right.

In Part II you can look up a disease or condition of special concern to you and read how The Four Aces and other free radical fighters can be of assistance in eliminating your discomfort and preventing a recurrence.

Finally, in Part III you can find the definition of new words, where to find a nutritionally trained physician, and how to research health information on your own.

It is my hope that with this information, you will be able to choose the very best ingredients, with a long and healthy life as a result.

—Carolyn Reuben

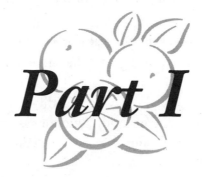

Part I

Antioxidants:
Nutritional Self-Defense

At this very moment a silent defense network circulates within and through every body cell as a united front against disease and deterioration. What it is and where its members come from varies, but they share one powerful aim: to neutralize dangerous fractions of oxygen known as free radicals. The following section describes both sides of the conflict: aggressors and defenders alike.

First, you'll be introduced to the wild ones within, the free radicals. Next, you'll meet The Four ACES, a team of free radical fighters whose members work better together than alone and which includes vitamin A (and its sidekick beta-carotene), vitamin C (and its partner, the bioflavonoids), vitamin E, and the mineral selenium.

Coenzyme Q10 (an enzyme), melatonin (a hormone), and cysteine (an amino acid) are also potent defenders of the realm within and are individually spotlighted.

Finally, you'll greet the Special Forces from the gardens of the world: bilberry, garlic, ginkgo biloba, green and black tea, and milk thistle.

Just when you thought staying healthy was so difficult, you'll discover that how well your body functions is greatly determined by how you answer one simple question: "What's cooking?"

The High Cost of Free Radicals

Imagine picking up a fine red apple from a bowl on the kitchen table. You slice it up and eat a piece. Then the phone rings, the clothes dryer goes off, and the mail arrives. Two hours later, you return to your apple. The slices left on your plate are brown. They have been attacked and spoiled by molecules of oxygen in the kitchen air, the same molecules that will rust the metal of automobiles. Since it is oxygen doing the dirty work, we say the apple and the car have been oxidized. The molecules doing the oxidizing are called oxidants.

Let's imagine you've left a bottle of cooking oil unrefrigerated in a hot kitchen for a week or two. When you use the oil, you'd probably smell or taste a difference and say the oil has gone rancid. This is another case of oxidants at work.

The medical term for oil or fat is *lipid*. Scientists call the process of fat turning rancid *lipid peroxidation*. Unfortunately, you have fat within every cell of your body, which Dr. Roy Walford, a UCLA gerontologist, terms "your own bodily butter," and there are times when you, too, turn rancid. The result can be as benign as wrinkled skin or as lethal as malignant cancer. How much damage results depends on many factors, including how long the reaction continues and in what tissue it occurs. It also depends on the

Free Radicals

What is it? A free radical is an unstable molecule, often a form of oxygen, that reacts with other molecules in a destructive way.

Why is it dangerous? Molecules are stable when they have pairs of electrons around their nucleus. When the number of electrons in a molecule is uneven, it is unstable, and that free radical steals an electron from another molecule to stabilize its own structure. The ensuing domino effect among molecules competing for electrons creates a tidal wave of electron thefts, causing damage and malfunction in the body. This theft of electrons is called *oxidation*. When it occurs in fat it is called *lipid peroxidation*.

How does it occur? Oxidation occurs inside the body during the normal process of metabolism. It is also caused by air pollution, radiation, cigarette smoke, sunlight, environmental chemicals, and exposure of metals and biological materials (including food) to oxygen.

What is the effect to your body? An excess of free radicals can cause different medical conditions, depending on which tissues are attacked. The free radicals may attack DNA

genetic predisposition, nutritional status, current health, and emotional stress level of the individual.

When the damage occurs in a blood vessel, it can initiate cardiovascular disease. When it happens to DNA, your unique genetic inheritance found within every cell nucleus, birth defects or cancer can result. When it happens to the lipids within the eye's crystalline lens, cataracts are formed. Thus, oxygen has earned the title "universal toxin"[1] and it seems the list of diseases and conditions caused by it just gets longer every day.

(your genetic inheritance) and cause cancer or birth defects; if they attack your pancreas, they can cause diabetes; in blood and blood vessels, they can cause cardiovascular disease; in the eye, they can cause cataracts. Often free radicals attack the fat within cell membranes. As a result, the membrane cannot properly select what enters and leaves the cell, making the cell dangerously vulnerable to toxins and further damage. Nonetheless, in low doses, free radicals are useful to the body: for example, they help kill bacteria.

What can you do to protect yourself? Antioxidants are nutritional substances that can stop free radicals from developing, can stop the cascade effect of numerous free radical reactions, and can repair damage caused by oxidation and lipid peroxidation. Antioxidants include vitamin A, carotenes (particularly beta-carotene and lycopene), vitamins C and E, the mineral selenium, bioflavonoids, amino acids such as cysteine and methionine, and herbs such as bilberry, garlic, milk thistle, and Ginkgo biloba.

What additional nutrients are needed? For antioxidants to work at their peak, the body needs adequate levels of zinc, copper, manganese, and vitamins B-5 and B-6.

Free Radicals Are to Blame

Oxidants are often free radicals. Free what? Chemists call the smallest unit that maintains its own uniqueness a *radical*. In your body, a free radical is "free" because it is missing an electron.

Perhaps you have seen a picture of an atom with something whirling around the nucleus. That something is an electron. Electrons are negatively charged particles that usually move in a fixed orbit around the nucleus of an atom.

Molecules are happiest when they have even pairs of electrons.

When a molecule is missing one electron, it is a free radical, and it eagerly and indiscriminately steals the electron it needs. Unfortunately, the victim of theft then becomes a free radical, and it immediately seeks an electron to steal, which will then create yet another free radical. Eventually there is a cascade of electron thefts, resulting in tissue damage. In addition, this explosive chain reaction creates new compounds which also contribute to the mess.

Just as the best place to pickpocket is in a crowd, so also the free radical prefers areas where lots of electrons congregate. Free radicals are especially partial to polyunsaturated fatty acids, which comprise about half of the fat content of the membrane surrounding every cell in your body.

Where Free Radicals Are Born

Free radicals are produced in the normal process of cell metabolism, which means the ordinary daily tasks of taking in nutrients, creating energy, reproducing, repairing damage, and shoveling out the trash left over from all the other functions. Free radicals are also produced in the body by alcohol, cured meats, artificial colorings, petrochemicals, inhaled fumes, herbicides, asbestos, smog, ultraviolet radiation, X rays, chemotherapy, smoking, exercise, emotional stress, physical trauma, some drugs, as well as other causes.

Usually, the body has ways to neutralize these free radicals on its own. Trouble results when more free radicals are produced than the body can neutralize.

The Body Protects Itself

When oxidation begins in living tissues, the body responds by creating substances to surround, control, and destroy the oxidants. These substances are called *antioxidants*. This being the case, you may be wondering why degenerative diseases occur at all. Why isn't damage always prevented by the vigilance of these internally generated antioxidants? Well, let's imagine a preschool with 30 three- and four-year-olds and only one teacher. The teacher is in the right place at the right time, but the poor lady is outnumbered and overpowered once the kids get going at full speed. She needs a staff of other adults around at all times! It's the same story in the battle against oxidation.

And so we come to the critical importance of a daily diet rich in fruits, vegetables, and whole grains: These foods act like the extra preschool staff, ensuring that oxidants perform their assigned functions and don't cause bedlam.

Free Radicals Aren't All Bad

What did I just mean by "assigned functions?" There is an ancient Chinese that says, "If Earth produced it, Heaven can find a use for it." We've painted free radicals as Public Enemy No. 1 thus far, but nature hates to waste anything, even a destructive force like free radicals. Oncologists, for example, use anthracycline antibiotics, which stimulate free radical production to fight cancer cells. Dr. Dean Black describes other endearing qualities of free radicals:

> An oxidant called nitric oxide helps control blood pressure, for example. When blood pressure goes up, cells in the vessel wall release nitric oxide, which causes the muscle layer to relax so that blood pressure goes back down. Heart-disease patients produce *less* nitric oxide, in fact, than healthy people do . . .[2]
>
> Nitric oxide also helps form memories. [According to S. Young,] "When (scientists) gave chicks a chemical that prevents cells from making nitric oxide and then trained them, the chicks rapidly forgot their lessons." Without nitric oxide, "the chick can learn the task but it can't retain the memory for it."[3]

Curiously, oxidants are used by our own immune system as a form of self-defense against invaders. When the invader approaches, our white blood cells bombard it with an *oxidative burst* of superoxide free radicals and hydrogen peroxide, overwhelming the enemy bacteria with oxidants until it dies.[4] This may be why a drug causing free radicals can be used against cancer cells. Although our own immune cells are destroyed in this process, others are created to take their place. A few of our soldiers are lost, but the war is won.

In fact, the superoxide free radical mentioned above is produced by the process of respiration (intake of oxygen, release of carbon dioxide) within the cells of our body.

"So," concludes Black, "the point isn't that oxidants are bad, merely that they must be carefully and precisely managed."[5] Like preschoolers.

The Antioxidant Defense System

Black crystallizes the various partners in this battle against free radical damage into what he calls the Antioxidant Defense System,[6] which protects us at four levels:

- First, it keeps oxidants from forming. It corrals oxygen into only those areas where it does us good, and keeps oxygen out of areas where it might do mischief. It also stops certain metals, like iron, from initiating oxidation. (Other metals involved in free radical production are copper, cadmium, mercury, and lead.)

- Second, the Antioxidant Defense System intercepts oxidants that manage to get formed, and puts the brake on chain reactions to stop the re-creation of numerous other oxidants.

- Third, it repairs damage caused by the oxidants that don't get intercepted.

- Fourth, it eliminates and replaces molecules that have been damaged beyond repair, and cleans up after itself, removing undesirable substances generated by its activities.

Working Together for the Common Good

The word *system* means individual elements functioning together as a whole. The term *Antioxidant Defense System* implies a close-knit interdependence, a team effort. The team players in this system include bacteria, enzymes, and nutrients.

Bacteria

Intestinal bacteria are not, themselves, considered antioxidants, but they decompose biochemical substances that can develop into oxidants. So, bacteria are part of our first line of defense.

Enzymes

Once oxidants do form, our second line of defense arrives. It's composed of enzymes—protein molecules that disarm some of the most dangerous oxidants before they start chain reactions.

"Enzymes," explains Elizabeth Somer, a registered dietician, "are like the equipment on an automobile production line; they speed the assembly process without becoming part of the car."[7] Although two substances might, given enough time, eventually bump into each other and react, an enzyme makes sure it happens, and happens quickly. For example, "a chemical reaction that might take hours or years to occur randomly will occur several thousand times in a split second with the aid of the enzyme."[8]

A good example of an enzyme antioxidant is *superoxide dismutase* (pronounced *super-oxide dis-mew-tays*). (In chemistry jargon, whenever you see the suffix *-ase* it indicates an enzyme.) Superoxide dismutase (SOD) can stop a chain reaction while it's happening. Thus, SOD is called a chain-breaking antioxidant. It does this by causing the oxidant called superoxide to dismute, or react with itself, and in doing so to disassemble into its less toxic individual parts. In this case, superoxide dismutes (disassembles) into hydrogen peroxide (which is a weaker oxidant) and oxygen.

Hydrogen peroxide isn't as dangerous as superoxide, but it's still toxic. Along comes our second important antioxidant enzyme, called *glutathione peroxidase* (*glue-ta-thigh-own per-ox-eh-days*). Glutathione peroxidase disassembles hydrogen peroxide into simple water and oxygen.[9] Glutathione peroxidase prevents the formation of free radicals.

Left alone, hydrogen peroxide will eventually react with itself and disassemble into water and oxygen, but this spontaneous transformation occurs slowly compared to what happens when glutathione peroxidase is present to spark the change.

Enzyme Helpers

Our body produces millions of enzymes, and each one of those enzymes has only one particular chemical reaction that is its responsibility. It may not do that job alone, however. Many enzymes have helpers, called *coenzymes* or *cofactors*. Many cofactors are nutrients. Antioxidant cofactors include selenium, copper, riboflavin, glutathione, coenzyme Q10, cysteine, manganese, zinc, and bioflavonoids. All these nutrients can be found in a diet rich in fruits, vegetables, and whole grains, and all are assistants essential to the antioxidant enzymes that protect our health.

For example, the mineral selenium is a coenzyme to glutathione peroxidase. In practical terms, this means if your diet is severely low in selenium, you aren't going to be having as much activity of the antioxidant enzyme glutathione peroxidase as you need, and you're going to have more free radical damage than you want.

When the body is low in manganese, zinc, or copper, not enough superoxide dismutase can be created to protect the body from free radical chain reactions and, again, damage occurs.[10]

I've mentioned that the body actually needs oxidants to perform some tasks. Enzymes serve as a second line in our antioxidant defense system by keeping already existing oxidants at low enough concentrations so that they can do the jobs assigned to them without proliferating into a wild, uncontrolled, and damaging chain reaction.

Nutrients

So, if the bacteria in our gut stop some oxidants from forming and certain enzymes keep already-formed oxidants under control, with coenzymes and cofactors lending a helping hand, what do we have in our body arsenal to get control of the situation when the number of oxidants reaches chain reaction stage and threatens us with significant damage?

If ever there was a good example of how we are provided by nature with a self-defense system organized to be as efficient as possible, here it is. Our third line of defense against damaging free radicals is as near to us as our next meal!

The Four Aces

Decades of research have clearly identified the following nutrients as strong and effective antioxidants: vitamins A, C, and E, and the mineral selenium. You can easily remember them as The Four ACES. Several other nutrients are also useful as part of the defense team, as are several herbs. I'll describe each, in turn, in the chapters that follow. I'll also suggest ways to include all of them in your daily diet.

You've got to admit we've got great teamwork going for us: One of the most remarkable aspects of this entire system is the intricate dance between the individual antioxidants themselves.

In the following chapters on The Four ACES, you'll discover how nature provides us with ways to maximize the use of whatever antioxidants we consume. Vitamin C regenerates vitamin E. The enzyme glutathione peroxidase regenerates a fatiguing vitamin C. Vitamin E protects the lipids in the bloodstream, while selenium is defending lipids in the cells and vitamin C is fighting free radicals in the watery areas of the body. Vitamin E fights free radicals where oxygen levels are high, and beta-carotene handles free radicals in areas where oxygen levels are low.

In other words, the interplay of The Four ACES is absolutely critical for the successful control of oxidants. We need to provide our bodies with not just one or two antioxidants, but with all of them for any of them to work optimally to protect us from old Janus-faced oxygen.

Notes

1. Attributed to French scientist Paul Bert in 1874, by Dean Black (1988), in *Taming Oxygen's Wild Side: How Antioxidants Guard Our Health* (p. 1). Springville, UT: Tapestry Press. [This excellent brochure can be ordered for $3.95 plus $1.00 shipping from Tapestry Press, 925 N. Main, Springville, UT 84663.]

2. Ibid., p.8.

3. Ibid., citing Young, S. (1993). The body's vital poison. *New Scientist* 137, 37.

4. Lonsdale, Derrick. (1986). Free oxygen radicals and disease. In *1986: A Year in Nutritional Medicine* (p. 89). New Canaan, CT: Keats.

5. Black, p. 8.

6. Ibid., p. 9.

7. Somer, Elizabeth. (1992). *The Essential Guide to Vitamins and Minerals* (p. 328). New York: HarperCollins.

8. Ibid.

9. Levine, Stephen A., and Kidd, Parris M. (1986). *Antioxidant Adaptation: Its Role in Free Radical Pathology* (p. 50). San Leandro, CA: Allergy Research Group.

10. Zidenberg-Cherr, Sheri, and Keen, Carl L. (1991). Essential trace elements in antioxidant processes. In *Trace Elements, Micronutrients and Free Radicals* (p. 127). Totowa, NJ: Humana.

〜〜 Vitamin A and Beta-Carotene

Vitamin A

In 1913, scientists isolated a vitamin for the very first time. Perhaps believing there would be no more than 26 vitamins in all, they named it vitamin A. In scientific language, vitamin A is called *retinol*, because it is found in the retina of all mammals. It is also found in the liver, which stores about 90 percent of the vitamin A found in the body of a reasonably well-nourished individual.

In 1928, enthusiastic researchers dubbed vitamin A the "anti-infective" vitamin, because of its ability to bolster our resistance to infections. More broadly, when you think of vitamin A, think of healthy linings. This vitamin is essential for the health and moisture of the skin and the specialized cells lining your eyes, nose, mouth, throat, lungs, esophagus, stomach, intestines, and urinary tract. These cells are called epithelial cells. When epithelial cells don't have as much vitamin A as they need, they thicken and harden.

For example, if you have a deficiency of vitamin A, you may see hardened small areas on the skin called keratoses. If you find

Vitamin A and Beta-Carotene

What are the functions of vitamin A? Vitamin A keeps skin moist and healthy. It also maintains the health of the inner linings of nose, throat, lungs, intestines, and urinary tract. It strengthens the immune system, promotes normal vision, and assures the proper development of the fetus.

What are the functions of beta-carotene? Beta-carotene converts to vitamin A in the body, yet maintains some immune system functions of its own: It protects against tumor development and helps create healthy sperm.

What are the signs of deficiency? Night blindness; susceptibility to infections; dry, scaly skin; hard, small bumps on upper arms; lack of appetite; dry eyes; dry, brittle hair with dandruff; frequent colds; weight loss; and the increased risk of cancer are all signs of a deficiency of vitamin A.

How is it absorbed into the bloodstream? Vitamin A is absorbed in the bloodstream through dietary fat.

What limits absorption? Liver damage, digestive diseases, mineral oil laxatives, drugs such as aspirin and Phenobarbital, air pollution, food additives, no-fat diet, and protein deficiency all limit absorption. People who have liver disease, diabetes, or low levels of thyroid hormone (hypothyroidism) have problems converting beta-carotene to vitamin A.

Where is it found? Preformed vitamin A is found in eggs, liver, fish oils, butter, milk, and cream. Beta-carotene is found in green, red, orange, or yellow fruits and vegetables.

Who are at risk of deficiency? Teens and others living on soda pop and fast food risk vitamin A and beta-carotene deficiencies, as do elderly living on tea, toast, and cereal, and people with cystic fibrosis or severe liver disease.

What are the signs of overdose? For preformed vitamin A, severe headaches, bone pain, dry rough skin, abdominal discomfort, vomiting, cracked lips, insomnia, fatigue, loss of body hair, brittle nails, night sweats, little or no menstruation, or birth defects are all signs of vitamin A overdose. For beta-carotene, the skin on the palms and soles of the feet turning a yellow-orange color signify an overdose.

What is the recommended daily allowance (RDA)? The RDA for preformed vitamin A is 375 micrograms (mcg) Retinol Equivalents (RE) for infants. (1 mcg of Retinol Equivalents is equal to 0.6 International Units [IU], so 375 mcg RE = 225 IU.) For children 1–3 years of age, it is 400 mcg RE (240 IU). For children 4–6, it is 500 mcg RE (300 IU). Children 7–10 need 700 mcg RE (420 IU). Males 11 and older require 1,000 mcg RE (600 IU), while females 11 and up and pregnant women should have 800 mcg RE (480 IU). Lactating women in months 1–6 need 1,300 mcg RE (780 IU), and those 6 months to 1 year require 1,200 mcg RE (720 IU). The RDA for beta-carotene for children is 3–5 mg; for adult men and women it is 10 mg.

What is the usual safe daily dose? Most adults can consume up to 20,000 IU of vitamin A, while children should be limited to 5,000 IU of vitamin A. However, individual sensitivity varies. For beta-carotene, the individual need for vitamin A dictates at what level the skin changes color. The dosages used in studies administering beta-carotene to people have ranged from 15 to 180 mg per day.

Warning on supplementation: A safe dosage of preformed vitamin A for pregnant women is 5,000 IU per day. What is excessive is an individual matter, but, in general, pregnant women should avoid consuming a total of more than 20,000 IU of preformed vitamin A per day.

As for beta-carotene, 10–20 mg per day is generally considered a safe dose, although the safest dose of all is to multiply the variety and quantity of red, yellow, and green fruits and vegetables in your diet rather than take a beta-carotene supplement. Eat a rainbow every day!

yourself catching one cold after another, it may mean the hardening has occurred inside your respiratory or digestive system. Here's why.

When your body is in good working order, a thin film of mucus inside the respiratory and digestive tracts latches on to foreign particles that might harm you if they hung around. Pulsating hair-like projections pass the particles upward and out in coughs or sneezes, or down and out through your bowel movements. If the lining of the respiratory or digestive system is thickened and hard, it cannot pulsate well enough to move potentially harmful particles away from your lungs in either direction, and you become more susceptible to infection.

Banking on the Liver

The liver serves as a vitamin A bank. When you eat vitamin A, it enters the body as retinol, and whatever retinol isn't immediately used by the body is changed to retinyl palmitate and stored in the liver. The liver holds on to these reserves of the vitamin, which you withdraw as needed. It takes about 3 months to use up the liver's reserves. Thus, if you are healthy, you don't have to consume vitamin A every single day to have an adequate supply, as long as you eat foods containing vitamin A regularly enough to replenish what has been used. However, the vitamin is used up more quickly when you are sick, have an infection, are injured, or are under severe emotional stress, so in these cases you need to increase your consumption through food sources or supplementation (see the discussion of beta-carotene, below).

The need for vitamin A varies with your age, stage of growth, calorie intake, physical exercise, pregnancy, and lactation. The vitamin is needed for proper cell differentiation and growth, so it is critically important in the formation of a fetus, and too little or too much vitamin A can have equally disastrous consequences.

Problems with Absorption

Vitamin A is a fat-soluble vitamin. That means if there was absolutely no fat or oil in your food, you couldn't pull vitamin A out of your intestines and into your bloodstream to be distributed to the body cells needing it. With all the publicity about eating a low-fat diet, this is a good reminder that nature works through the Golden Mean, and some fat, about 5 grams a day, is necessary for adequate vitamin A absorption.

Since absorption of vitamin A depends on absorption of fat through the intestinal wall, diseases and conditions that interrupt the normal function of either the intestines or the liver (which produces essential digestive enzymes) will interfere with vitamin A absorption. Some of these conditions include celiac disease (an inherited sensitivity to the gluten in wheat), Crohn's disease (an inflammation of the intestinal tract), obstruction of the gall bladder, infectious hepatitis, and jaundice.

Vitamin A absorption is also affected by the amount of protein in your diet. Fat-soluble vitamins don't mix well with the watery element of blood, just as oil and water don't easily mix when you make salad dressing. When you need to use the vitamin A stored in your liver, that stored form of vitamin A is carried in the bloodstream a special protein called a "retinol-binding protein." Consequently, protein deficiency can make symptoms of vitamin A deficiency worsen.

Vitamin A also needs the mineral zinc to perform its work, so a deficiency of zinc will lower the productivity of vitamin A, even if enough vitamin A is available.

The use of mineral oil as a laxative will pull any fat-soluble vitamin, including vitamin A, into the oil and out of the intestine, contributing to vitamin A deficiency. Some other causes of poor vitamin A absorption include certain drugs, such as aspirin and barbiturates like Phenobarbital,[1] sodium benzoate and other food additives, and air pollutants.

Sources of Vitamin A

You can tell vitamin A is a very important nutrient because sources for it are so widely distributed in both the animal and plant kingdoms. Vitamin A is in egg yolks, dairy products (like butter, milk, and cream), animal livers, and fish oils. These animal sources provide ready-made, preformed vitamin A, or retinol. Plants offer something called beta-carotene, also referred to as *provitamin A* because your body uses beta-carotene to create vitamin A in just the amount needed at that time.

Beta-Carotene

There are at least 500 carotenes (a family of red-orange compounds found in food of various kinds), but only about 50 have biological importance to humans and animals, and of these the most important is beta-carotene. One molecule of beta-carotene converts into two molecules of vitamin A. This transformation occurs in the intestines. The vitamin A is then transported in the lymph and bloodstream to the liver, where it is stored. However, unconverted beta-carotene is also stored in the body, mostly in fat, but also in lesser amounts in the liver, adrenals, skin, ovaries, and testes. Until recently, little attention was paid to beta-carotene except as a precursor to vitamin A. Recent research is giving the nutrient more of its own starring role as an antioxidant. We now know that beta-carotene acts as a therapeutic agent with biological effects all its own.

Back in 1985, for example, researchers at Hoffman-La Roche Inc. discovered that beta-carotene enhances the work of the immune system in addition to its vitamin A activity.[2] Also in 1985, another study found that beta-carotene, along with several carotenes that do not convert to vitamin A, was able to protect the skin of experimental animals from ultraviolet-light-induced tumor formation as well as from tumors induced by chemicals.[3] In addition, beta-carotene is an excellent defense against a toxic form of oxygen produced by our bodies called "singlet oxygen." So, adequate levels of beta-carotene and other carotenes are important for our well-being in addition to their vitamin A activity.

Sources of Beta-Carotene

Your best sources of beta-carotene are carrots, papayas, sweet potatoes, collard greens, spinach, and other dark-green leafy vegetables, as well as cantaloupe and winter squash, including pumpkin. Asparagus, peppers, corn, peas, beans, and cauliflower also contain beta-carotene, as do oranges, nectarines, mangos, figs, grapes, cranberries, apricots, strawberries, and watermelon. Some beta-carotene is also found in fish, shellfish, and dairy products such as milk, butter, cheese, and ice cream.

Some Limiting Factors

Beta-carotene in produce is easily destroyed when exposed to light and oxygen. The more we manipulate fruits and vegetables in preparing them for the table, the more beta-carotene is lost. The nutrient also disappears during storage and when exposed to moisture and heat.

Beta-carotene converts to vitamin A in the intestines, with the help of protein and digestive enzymes called bile salts. Inadequate digestive enzymes or a protein-deficient diet can therefore limit the amount of vitamin A able to be produced.

Too little thyroid hormone (thyroxine) can also reduce the absorption of beta-carotene, and in that way reduce vitamin A levels.

Dangers of Over-Use

Preformed vitamin A, or retinol, can build up in the liver until a level is reached where severe headaches, joint pain, cracked, dry lips, brittle nails, night sweats, insomnia, and falling hair result. Fatigue, abdominal discomfort, little or no menstruation, constipation, bulging eyeballs, and swollen hands and feet have also been reported. Most tragically, women who have, during the first trimester of pregnancy, taken 13-*cis*-retinoic acid (isotretinoin), a form of vitamin A prescribed for acne (and sometimes taken surreptitiously to improve an aging complexion), have given birth to babies with birth defects, including malformation of the face, skull, jaw, heart, or central nervous system. Birth defects have occurred when the drug has been taken for from 1 to 7 weeks, beginning during the first 10 weeks after conception. Please note: Women who have stopped taking 13-*cis*-retinoic acid (trademarked as Retin-A) at least one month prior to conception probably do not have to worry about the drug affecting their fetus, particularly if they have practiced contraception at least 1 month before and 1 month after taking Retin-A.[4]

A safe dosage of preformed vitamin A for a pregnant woman, or a woman anticipating pregnancy, is 5,000 IU per day. For the rest of us, signs of toxicity usually occur only at chronic, daily doses of over 50,000 IU for adults, or 20,000 IU for children. A dose generally recognized as safe is 10,000 IU per day, though some people with low vitamin A stores in their liver can take much more without harm.

All the signs and symptoms of vitamin A excess except birth defects are easily corrected by cutting back or stopping consumption of vitamin A.

One unpleasant side effect of consuming too much beta-carotene is a yellowish-orange discoloration of the hands and feet. This effect has occurred after taking 30 mg or more per day, depending on the level of vitamin A already stored in the liver and the body's need for the vitamin. The color fades as soon as you stop or cut back the dosage, and there is no harm in this color change. You can instantly tell if you have jaundice (a skin yellowing which indicates a liver disorder) instead of too much beta-carotene in your system: jaundice turns the whites of your eyes yellow, while with excessive beta-carotene the whites of your eyes are still white.

Recently, a well-designed study published in the *New England Journal of Medicine* suggested that beta-carotene supplements increased the risk of lung cancer among smokers.[5] This has confounded the scientific community, since over a dozen intervention trials in nine countries have been funded, using dosages ranging from 15 mg to 180 mg per day, and this is the first with such negative results. As a supplement, beta-carotene has been taken by many individuals for as long as 15 years, at doses of 30 to 180 mg, without adverse effects.[6] The general consensus is a wait-and-see attitude, because results from additional trials are due within the next 5 years. It is hoped that their results will clarify what is now a confusing situation. Supplement beta-carotene modestly, if at all, until this issue is resolved, using only 3–20 mg (5,000–33,333 IU) of beta-carotene per day. One carrot can contain 7,900 IU of beta-carotene, 1 cup of dried apricots 14,000 IU,[7] and one medium stalk of broccoli can contain 4,500 IU, so a diet rich in produce is very rich in beta-carotene.

Measuring Units

Vitamin A is measured in International Units, as are all oil-based vitamins (vitamins A, E, and K). One IU of vitamin A equals 0.3 micrograms (mcg) of retinol, or 0.6 mcg of beta-carotene. (As mentioned in the section above on beta-carotene, one molecule of beta-carotene forms two molecules of vitamin A.)

So, if your antioxidant formula states "2 tablets contain 50,000 IU beta-carotene," how many milligrams of beta-carotene are you consuming? First, 0.6 mcg is the same as 0.0006 mg, so, 1 IU equals 0.0006 mg. Second, since your formula contains 50,000 IU, multiply 0.0006 by 50,000. The answer is 30 mg of beta-carotene. (If your beta-carotene has 30,000 IU in it, multiply 0.0006 by 30,000; you are taking 18 mg of beta-carotene.)

Sometimes, the relationship of beta-carotene and preformed vitamin A is expressed according to their relative biological activity: Because beta-carotene is less well-absorbed from the intestine than is retinol, and its biological activity decreases as intake increases, a Retinol Equivalent (RE) was created so that 6 mcg of beta-carotene equal 1 mcg of retinol. That means 1 IU is equal to 0.6 RE.

Conclusion

Vitamin A is crucial for healthy skin, an active immune system, a well-functioning respiratory tract, and proper development of the fetus. In the form of beta-carotene in fruits and vegetables, it seems to help protect us against cancer. It is an important collaborator in an antioxidant defense team. For adequate levels of this vitamin, eat a rainbow of foods daily, emphasizing a wide variety of fresh, colorful fruits and vegetables, whole grains, and seafoods.

Notes

1. Leo, Maria Anna, et al. (1984). Decreased hepatic vitamin A after drug administration in men and in rats. *American Journal of Clinical Nutrition* 40, 1131–1136.

2. Shapiro, S., and Bendich, A. (1985). Effect of dietary carotenoids on lymphocyte responses to mitogens. *Federal Proceedings* 44, 544.

3. Kornhauser, A., et al. (1985). Effect of dietary beta-carotene on psoralen-induced phototoxicity. *Annals of the New York Academy of Science* 453, 91–104.

4. Olin, Bernie R., ed. (1994). *Facts and Comparisons* (p. 543d). Facts and Comparisons Inc.: St. Louis.

5. The Alpha-Tocopherol, Beta Carotene Cancer Prevention Study Group. (1994). The effect of vitamin E and beta carotene on the incidence of lung cancer and other cancers in male smokers. *The New England Journal of Medicine* 330(15), 1029–1035.

6. Bendich, Adrienne. (1988). The safety of beta-carotene. *Nutrition and Cancer* 11, 207–214.

7. Robertson, Laurel. (1993). *Laurel's Kitchen* (pp. 465–469). Berkeley, CA: Ten Speed Press.

≈⊘ Vitamin C and Bioflavonoids

North Americans consume vitamin C more often than any other nutritional supplement.[1] The vitamin became associated in the public mind with improved health after the 1970 publication of *Vitamin C and the Common Cold* by two-time Nobel Prize winner Linus Pauling.

Pauling's book sparked a heated controversy over the benefits of taking large doses of this single vitamin. Opponents claim vitamin C simply will not prevent colds, and is unnecessary in large doses. Proponents say the vitamin is outstandingly effective, but only if you take large enough doses. For example, Dr. Robert F. Cathcart III, a physician in Los Altos, California, recommends 30–60 *grams* (remember, 1 gram = 1,000 mg) of vitamin C for a mild cold, with doses spread over 24 hours.[2]

Aside from the common cold controversy, vitamin C boasts numerous benefits that are not so hotly debated. Curing scurvy, for example. Vitamin C's biological name is ascorbic acid; ascorbic is Latin for "without scurvy." Among Europeans, the first recorded cure of scurvy with vitamin C was in 1535, when a Canadian native from Quebec promised French explorer Jacques Cartier that his crew's deadly disease would disappear if they consumed an herbal remedy made from a local tree. One source

23

Vitamin C and Bioflavonoids

What are the functions of vitamin C? Vitamin C serves as a key link within important enzyme chain reactions. It also regenerates vitamin E; forms and protects collagen (the protein holding body cells together); helps the immune system function well; regulates blood sugar; protects the eye from damage by ultraviolet light; keeps cholesterol from forming plaque on artery walls; prevents blood clots; improves lung function; makes iron more absorbable in the intestines; prevents the transformation of nitrites (a food preservative) into cancer-causing nitrosamines; and is involved in the creation of hormones that regulate stress and inflammation, including adrenalin and corticosteroids.

What are the functions of bioflavonoids? Numerous functions have been reported for the bioflavonoids, yet research is often conflicting and is, therefore, controversial. Some reports claim bioflavonoids can strengthen capillary walls; reduce inflammation; fight viruses, bacteria, and fungi; detoxify carcinogens; alleviate "hot flashes"; reduce the risk of cataract in people with diabetes; protect vitamin C from destruction; reduce histamine response in allergic reactions; prevent spontaneous abortion; reduce ulceration; and reduce the risk of stroke.

What are the signs of deficiency? When vitamin C (also called ascorbic acid) intake is below 10 milligrams (mg) per day, a deficiency disease called *scurvy* appears. Many of the following symptoms of borderline ascorbic acid deficiency appear in the general public even without frank cases of scurvy: dry skin, bleeding gums, poor wound healing, small hemorrhages under the skin, weakness, muscle cramps, tender joints, loss of appetite, depression, and increased susceptibility to infection and disease.

A deficiency in bioflavonoids is often characterized by bleeding gums, varicose veins, hot flashes during menopause, easy bruising, small pinpoint red blotches under the skin, nosebleeds, and hemorrhoids.

How is vitamin C absorbed into the bloodstream? Vitamin C is absorbed through fluids in the diet.

What limits absorption? Your state of health is the limiting factor in absorption. Interestingly, the stronger and deeper the infection, traumatic condition (such as a burn), or disease, the more vitamin you can absorb.

Who is at risk of deficiency? Those who eat less than nine fruit and vegetable servings a day (1 serving equals ½ cup of chopped, raw, or cooked vegetables or 1 cup of leafy raw vegetables; 1 piece of fruit or melon wedge; ¾ cup juice; ½ cup canned fruit, or ¼ cup dried fruit[3]); those who are ill, emotionally stressed, traumatized by a burn other injury, or who have congestive heart failure; those who live in a polluted environment; those who smoke tobacco or marijuana; those who work at a physically demanding job; those who work in extremely hot temperatures and sweat a great deal; those who use oral contraceptives; those who eat institutional food or other food prepared and stored for long periods of time; and those infants who are fed exclusively cow's milk are all at risk of a deficiency of vitamin C.

What are the sources for vitamin C? Vitamin C is found in citrus fruits, tomatoes, strawberries, cabbage, green leafy vegetables (kale, parsley, collards, mustard greens, chard), green peppers, broccoli, cantaloupe, cauliflower, asparagus, and baked potatoes.

What are the sources for bioflavonoids? The sources of bioflavonoids are similar to those of vitamin C: citrus fruits, grapes, plums, black currants, apricots, buckwheat, cherries, blackberries, apples, tea, and onions.

What are the signs of overdose? Diarrhea or abdominal cramping are frequently reported signs of vitamin C overdose.

> **What is the Recommended Dietary Allowance (RDA)?**
> For vitamin C, the RDA for infants birth to 6 months old is 30
> mg, for infants 7 months to 1 year it is 35 mg. For children 1 to
> 3 years old it is 40 mg, for those 4 to 10 years of age it is 45 mg,
> and for 11 to 14 year olds it is 50 mg. For most people over 15
> years of age, the RDA is 60 mg. For those who are pregnant, 70
> mg is recommended. Nursing mothers require 95 mg during
> the first 6 months, while those in the second 6 months need 90
> mg. Cigarette smokers require 100 mg. There is no RDA estab-
> lished for bioflavonoids.
>
> **What is the usual safe daily dose?** One way to find your

claims it was the Anneda pine, another the yellow cedar tree.
Whatever the tree, according to the ship's log which Cartier later
published, the captain was told "to take the bark and leaves of the
said tree, and boil it together, then to drink of the said decoction
one day, and the other not, and the dreggs [sic] of it to be put upon
his legs that is sick."[4]

Scurvy progresses from small hemorrhages under the skin and
bleeding gums to joint pain and swelling, falling teeth, ulcers in
the mouth, anemia, and severe weakness leading to death. Having
nothing to lose but the rest of his crew, Cartier found two men
willing to try the tree brew. Within a week their condition had
clearly improved, and the others clamored over each other to par-
take of the liquid miracle. Cartier's expedition in the Gulf of St.
Lawrence was saved.

Unfortunately, some 200 years passed (and with them thousands of sailors) before James Lind, a British naval physician,
compared six different purported cures for scurvy and discovered
that citrus fruits did the job best. Even so, it took 48 more years
and still more deaths before the British admiralty agreed to provide all their sailors with lime juice (ergo the nickname "limey")
and 118 years for the British Board of Trade to require the same
for all merchant ship crews.[5]

proper dose is to keep taking more vitamin C until you experience diarrhea, then reduce your next dose a small amount. This is called "taking vitamin C to bowel tolerance." When you are healthy, that dose will be strikingly lower than when you are ill. In general, the vitamin serves as an antioxidant at levels of at least 150 mg per day. For bioflavonoids, your dose should be around 1,000 mg per day.

Warning on supplementation: Over time, chewable vitamin C tablets can destroy the enamel on your teeth. Use these tablets only occasionally, never as your primary source of the vitamin.

Healing with Vitamin C

Each of The Four ACES has numerous benefits in the human body, some related to their ability to subdue free radicals and some based on other mechanisms of action. Vitamin C's power over scurvy, for example, is not specifically due to control over free radicals. Likewise, other mechanisms of action allow the vitamin to help heal wounds; to serve as an excellent antihistamine; to alleviate hay fever; to control the growth of bones, teeth, gums, blood vessels, and ligaments; to reduce the sensation of pain; to improve iron absorption; to help create sex hormones and the hormones that control our reaction to stress; to help regulate our moods; to form collagen (the connective tissue that holds our body together); and to fight both viruses and bacteria.

As a free radical scavenger, vitamin C keeps many different parts of us humming like a well-tuned motor. Robert A. Jacob, in a 1991 article in *The American Journal of Clinical Nutrition*, lists some of vitamin C's amazing feats as an antioxidant: Vitamin C prevents cardiovascular disease by protecting blood fats from being oxidized and transformed into dangerous plaque along artery walls. The vitamin protects the eyes from oxidation, helping prevent cataracts, macular degeneration, and other assaults on sight. It also protects sperm from oxidative damage that can lead

ility or dangerous mutations in a child who is conceived.[6]
Vitamin C protects us against many forms of cancer. As an example, the presence of an adequate amount of vitamin C in the stomach stops nitrites from forming nitrosamine compounds, which are the cause of oral and gastric cancers among smokers, tobacco chewers, and others exposed to high levels of nitrites, possibly including children exposed to too many hot dogs.

In June 1994, a University of Southern California epidemiology team reported finding a greater risk of childhood leukemia in children eating more than 12 hot dogs a month.[7] Other reports in the same Harvard University publication, called *Cancer Causes and Control*, found a higher rate of brain tumors among children whose fathers generally ate more than 12 hot dogs a month. The greatest risk was among children whose fathers usually ate an average of 23 hot dogs a month and among children who ate around 19 hot dogs a month. The researchers suggested that the nitrites used to preserve hot dogs might be to blame. They were quick to point out, by the way, that their study hadn't focused on the hot dog–cancer connection, but the correlation appeared in their statistics so prominently it couldn't be ignored. There may well be some other explanation that will be revealed in future research. Nevertheless, since vitamin C stops the transformation of nitrites into carcinogenic nitrosamines, if you're serving hot dogs for lunch, be sure you and your children drink orange juice or tomato juice, eat foods rich in vitamin C along with the meal, or swallow a vitamin C supplement with those grilled dogs. (See the chapter entitled "Tea" for green tea's similar talent at protecting you from nitrosamine formation.)

Adriamycin is a drug used effectively against many kinds of cancer, but the drug is so strong it damages the heart, possibly through peroxidation of the lipids in heart tissue. Vitamin C was given to guinea pigs with cancer who were being treated with adriamycin and effectively prevented damage to the animals' hearts.[8]

As an antioxidant, vitamin C is a team player. While vitamin E shines wherever there is fat and oil, vitamin C reigns supreme in the body's water element. Researchers believe the two vitamins work synergistically, meaning they function well together. Vitamin

E is used up as it fights free radicals. In its fatigued form, it becomes toxic to the body; but when vitamin C is present, the vitamin C regenerates the fatigued form of vitamin E, in effect recycling it so the vitamin E can keep after free radicals. Thus, enough vitamin C in body tissues assures adequate levels of vitamin E as well.[9]

Vitamin C, too, becomes used up in the process of protecting the body and regenerating vitamin E. So the body, ever the conservationist, arranges for vitamin C to be regenerated by the enzyme glutathione peroxidase (and, yes, glutathione peroxidase is regenerated by yet another substance).

Symptoms Of Marginal Deficiency

There's a wide spectrum of symptoms possible between mild vitamin C deficiency and outright scurvy. Count how many of the following symptoms of marginal vitamin C deficiency you can claim as your own:

- Irritability, anxiety, or depression
- Weight loss
- Loose teeth
- Bleeding gums
- Loss of appetite
- Limb pain or tender joints
- Dry skin
- Poor wound healing
- Small hemorrhages under the skin
- Weakness
- Muscle cramps
- Increased susceptibility to infections and disease

If you suffer from several of these symptoms, you may need to change your eating habits. An easy way to add vitamin C to your daily diet is to consume more fresh fruits and vegetables. The U.S. Department of Agriculture recommends nine fruit and vegetable servings *each day* for optimum health (see the box above for serving sizes).

Here are some suggestions for achieving this goal: Snack on sweet slices of citrus fruit, and remember exotic varieties such as kiwis; make large baked potatoes the focus of several lunches, varying the trimmings; add chopped purple cabbage, parsley, or cilantro to a green salad; pour some Caesar or ranch salad dressing into a small cup and dip raw or cooked vegetables into it (even fussy children tend to love veggies this way).

Dosage

Vitamin C is essential for life, yet humans, apes, monkeys, and guinea pigs are unique among the animals of the world in not being able to produce this substance for ourselves. Scientists think we lost the ability to create vitamin C from glucose some 60 million years ago. This means we are dependent on our food supply for our daily vitamin C.

It takes only about 10 milligrams (mg) of vitamin C a day, the amount of the vitamin found in one banana or one swallow of orange juice, to prevent the loose teeth and bleeding gums of scurvy. But, researchers like Emanual Cheraskin, a physician, dentist, author of scientific papers and books on clinical nutrition, and professor emeritus at the University of Alabama Medical Center in Birmingham, point out that "vitamin C influences every tissue and organ in the body," and that we may need more of the nutrient for optimum functioning than the minimum dose that will prevent scurvy.[10]

"Our paleolithic ancestors," notes Mark Levine of the National Institutes of Health, "were estimated to have consumed 400 mg of vitamin C per day and a diet containing 1 gram (1,000 mg) per day in foods is not difficult to achieve today."[11] The Recommended Dietary Allowances (RDA, that level the government has set, with what they consider a comfortable margin for biochemical individuality) for vitamin C is far below these figures, at just 60 mg for most adults.

You will notice in the box at the beginning of this chapter that if you smoke, if you are pregnant, or if you are nursing a baby, the RDA is greater than 60 mg daily. Other conditions necessitating an increase in your daily intake of vitamin C, which are not mentioned in the RDAs, include serious burns; rheumatic fever; using the birth control pill; congestive heart failure; thrombophlebitis; anemia; diarrhea; rheumatoid arthritis; living in a polluted city; surgery; infections of any kind; injury; diseases of the kidney, liver, stomach, or intestines; and cancer.

Cheraskin suggests if you choose to be "abnormal" and opt for fewer than two colds a year, a lower than 40 percent chance of hemorrhoids, and a lower than 30 percent chance of high cholesterol, then you will need more than the government's recommended dose. In fact, Cheraskin believes that most Americans need between 2 and 10 grams (2,000–10,000 mg) daily. Levine, too, notes that "on a mg/kg basis, all animals that synthesize ascorbic acid make at least 10-fold more than the human RDA. Primates in captivity require about 10–20-fold more than the human RDA on a weight-adjusted basis to maintain health."[12]

A reasonable middle ground may be not to take anyone's word for it, but to find your own unique need for the vitamin. The method for this is called "taking C to bowel tolerance." It is a technique developed by Dr. Cathcart, who began taking vitamin C to cure his own hay fever, and then discovered, beginning in 1970, that he could take a dose of vitamin C when he was ill that he couldn't tolerate when he was well. Applying this discovery to his patients, he found that the sicker his patients were, the more vitamin C they could tolerate before diarrhea occurred (see Table 1 on the following page). Anxiety, exercise, severe temperatures, and emotional stress also increased the amount of vitamin C his patients could tolerate before suffering digestive symptoms.

Taking vitamin C to bowel tolerance means you are the ultimate judge when you have taken enough, for as soon as you take so much you feel stomach cramps or diarrhea, you cut back each subsequent dose a few grams until you don't experience bowel disturbance. That is your optimum dose at that time.

Over the past 24 years, Cathcart has found the usual bowel tolerance doses for vitamin C, which all are given in from 4 to 25 divided doses over one 24-hour period, stretch from 4 to 15 grams for a normal healthy individual to 150–200+ grams for those with mononucleosis.[13]

Cathcart points out that if you have the flu and your body

Table 1 Usual Bowel Tolerance Doses

Condition	Grams per 24 hr	Doses per 24 hr
Normal	4–15	4
Mild cold	30–60	6–10
Severe cold	60–10	8–15
Influenza	100–150	8–20
Coxsackievirus	100–150	8–20
Mononucleosis	150–200	12–25
Viral pneumonia	100–200+	12–25
Hay fever, asthma	15–20	4–8
Environmental and food allergies	.05–50	4–8
Burn, injury, surgury	25–150	4–6
Anxiety, exercise, or other mild stresses	15–25	4–6
Cancer	15–100	4–15
Ankylosing spondylitis	15–100	5–15
Reiter's syndrome	15–60	4–15
Acute anterior uveitis	30–100	4–15
Rheumatoid arthritis	15–100	4–25
Bacterial infections	30–200+	10–25
Infectious hepatitis	3–100	6–15
Candida infections	15–200+	6–25

From Cathcart, Robert F., III. (1981). Vitamin C, titrating to bowel tolerance, *anascorbemia*, and acute induced scurvy. *Medical Hypothesis* 7, 1360–1361. Used with permission.

requires 100 grams of vitamin C to combat it, if you only consume 10 or even 20 grams (which may seem to you an outrageously high dose), not much will happen. Yet, if you keep taking the vitamin to bowel tolerance, 90 percent of your symptoms can disappear within a day or two.[14]

Don't Stop Suddenly

If you have taken vitamin C to bowel tolerance for a number of days, *don't* suddenly stop taking the vitamin supplement once your symptoms have vanished. If you do, your body will convert the vitamin C in your bloodstream into other biochemicals. You'll be left with a severe deficiency of the nutrient, which can lead to a relapse of the same infection or the development of a new infection.[15]

The proper way to come off high doses of vitamin C is to do so *slowly*, reducing your dosage only to your bowel tolerance level. You will find that this level decreases day by day as you recover from your illness, until you are entirely well and can return to your normal protective dose or can rely on a wholesome diet alone.

Protect Your C

When your diet is rich in fruits and vegetables, you are providing your cells an on-going supply of vitamin C. This is necessary because vitamin C is water soluble, and is quickly eliminated in the urine.

By the time it is cooked, particularly cooked in water, a food that was originally rich in the vitamin may have only a meager amount left. Vitamin C also disappears due to warm temperatures, exposure to oxygen, and the passage of time after produce is picked. For example, in the course of their journey from the soil of Idaho to supermarkets in New York City, potatoes lose as much as 60 percent of their vitamin C content. By the time you mash them, hash them, bake them, or boil them, another 40 to 50 percent of their remaining vitamin C content has vanished.[16]

Transportation, storage, cooking, and serving are only four of a total of 30 links in the chain from garden to gullet, says Cheraskin, and at every link the nutritional content of food diminishes until after one hour on a restaurant buffet, "you might as well nibble on the steam table."[17]

Sources of Vitamin C

Most fruits and vegetables provide some vitamin C, but particularly good sources are citrus fruits (oranges, grapefruits, tangerines, lemons), tomatoes, strawberries, cabbage, green leafy vegetables (kale, parsley, collard and mustard greens, chard), green peppers, broccoli, cantaloupe, cauliflower, asparagus, and baked potatoes.

Toxicity

Vitamin C is one of the safest supplements you can take, but even C has its hazards for some people, at some doses.

Dental erosion. Patricia Hausman, author of *The Right Dose: How to Take Vitamins & Minerals Safely*, points out a common mistake that can have devastating consequences: chewable vitamin C supplements destroy the enamel (the outer surface) of teeth![18] Sucking and chewing on sweet vitamin C tablets once in a while won't cause the damage, but if you're in the habit of chewing your vitamin C each day, it may take only a few months before you find your teeth becoming sensitive when you brush, or worse, needing full crowns. Swallow your vitamin C in ordinary tablet form and you won't have to worry about a dental disaster.

Kidney stones. All of us change some of the vitamin C in our bodies into a biochemical called both oxalic acid and oxalate. Some people can take a high dose of vitamin C and not produce extra oxalate, while others produce excessive amounts of oxalate, not only from vitamin C, but also from oxalate-containing foods, from a deficiency of magnesium, calcium, vitamins B-6 or B-1, inadequate water consumption, or other factors. In any case, oxalate in the urine doesn't bother people. Oxalate in the form of a calcium–oxalate stone lodged in a kidney, on the other hand, is excruciatingly painful. People who create kidney stones are prone to do so even if they don't consume vitamin C. They might want to consume less than 1,000 mg of vitamin C per day, just to be safe. In addition, anyone with previous kidney disease might want to consult a nutritionally trained medical professional who can recommend safe dosages of vitamin C and other supplements.

There are also reasons why vitamin C might actually reduce

kidney stone formation: the vitamin is a diuretic, causing increased urine flow; it acidifies the urine, reducing the combination of calcium and oxalate; and it binds calcium, which also prevents the creation of a calcium–oxalate stone.[19]

Finding references in the medical literature to people actually producing kidney stones because of taking vitamin C supplements is fairly rare. Nevertheless, if you have a history of kidney stones or learn from laboratory tests that your body produces excessive oxalic acid, consult a physician with experience using vitamin C before taking supplements of the vitamin.

Excess iron. For decades, medical authorities have urged Americans to consume more iron. The problem with getting enough iron is not only that we eat too little of the mineral, it's also that the mineral is very difficult for the body to absorb, so not all that we eat gets into the bloodstream where it does us good.

One of vitamin C's uses is to increase iron absorption. This is of benefit to everyone except those who have a genetic predisposition to absorb *too much* iron, a condition called hemochromatosis. People with hemochromatosis should not take supplements of vitamin C.[20] To be safe, before you take large doses of vitamin C, check with a medical professional familiar with your health history to make sure you don't have this or any other condition that causes increased iron absorption.

Bioflavonoids as C's Helpers

In the 1930s, Dr. Albert Szent-Gyorgyi, the Nobel Prize–winning Hungarian chemist who first synthesized vitamin C, still had an unpurified supply of C on hand when someone with a bleeding problem needed help. The scientist provided some of his vitamin preparation, and the bleeding stopped. By the time he was asked to help with the same problem again, he had purified and isolated ascorbic acid, but this C didn't work.

Szent-Gyorgyi investigated his old, "impure" preparation, and discovered within it something which, he wrote, "promptly cured the bleedings."[21] He called the substance vitamin P, but in the 1950s the American scientific community rejected that designation because they could not prove the substance was essential for life. The curious substance turned out to be a large family of substances which became known as flavones or flavonoids. There are over 500 different "flavonoids" but not all of them are biologically active. "Bio" flavonoids signifies those family members that influence animal and human bodies in some way.

To this day, no specific dietary need for bioflavonoids has been established, and so you won't find them in the RDAs. Nevertheless, research over the past 60 years suggests they are useful for a range of conditions. They are definitely antioxidants, and in fact they have been identified as the major antioxidant in the average Western diet.[22] As an antioxidant, bioflavonoids protect the liver from damage by industrial chemicals and viral hepatitis.[23]

Bioflavonoids protect vitamin C from being destroyed. They strengthen capillary walls, and therefore help prevent stroke, hemorrhoids, varicose veins, nosebleeds, bruising, bleeding gums, and pinpoint red blotches beneath the skin called petechiae. Because of their ability to strengthen blood vessel walls, they also seem capable of preventing hot flashes during menopause.

Bioflavonoids also inhibit the development of cancer, possibly by protecting DNA from damage[24] and by altering dangerous substances so they cannot be absorbed into the bloodstream from the gastrointestinal tract.[25]

Flavonoids have been used for eye conditions with great success. Dr. Alan R. Gaby in Pikesville, Maryland, and Dr. Jonathan V. Wright in Kent, Washington, have used a combination of nutrients, including bioflavonoids, to treat both macular degeneration and cataracts.[26]

The Chinese have used ginkgo biloba and other flavonoid-containing herbs for rheumatoid arthritis for centuries. This is understandable, since animal research has found that flavonoids provide pain relief and reduce inflammation.[27]

Flavonoids seem to work synergistically with vitamin C for allergy relief. In one study published in the *Journal of Allergy and Clinical Immunology* in 1992, flavonoids added to a solution of ascorbic acid significantly stopped the release of histamine from white blood cells of allergic individuals.[28]

Sources of Bioflavonoids

When you peel an orange, if you carefully remove the white stuff stuck to the fruit, you're denying yourself one of the most convenient sources of bioflavonoids, the white rind of citrus fruit. In addition, bioflavonoids are found in grapes, plums, black currants, apricots, buckwheat, cherries, blackberries, apples, tea, and onions.

Dosage of Bioflavonoids

In general, 500–1,000 mg of bioflavonoids per day will enhance the body's use of vitamin C and provide you with the benefits that are bioflavonoids' own unique gifts.

Conclusion

Vitamin C and bioflavonoids work both singly and synergistically to keep the body physically together and running smoothly and efficiently. The influence of these antioxidant nutrients on your immune system and numerous other systems is so pervasive that even minor signs of deficiency are best corrected quickly.

Notes

1. Jonas, Gabrielle. (1993). Vitamin and mineral supplements: What Americans are taking. *Medical Tribune*, April 29, p. 5.
2. Cathcart, Robert F., III, (1981). Vitamin C, titrating to bowel tolerance, anascorbemia, and acute induced scurvy. *Medical Hypothesis* 7, 1359–1376.
3. USDA Human Nutrition Information Services, June 8, 1994.
4. Cartier, Jacques (translated by John Florio). *Navigations to Newe Fraunce* (pp. 64–68). Ann Arbor, MI: Ann Arbor University Microfilms Inc. March of American Facsimile Series Number 10.
5. Castleman, Michael. (1987). *Cold Cures* (p. 92). New York: Ballantine.
6. Jacob, Robert A., et al. (1991). Immunocompetence and oxidant defense during ascorbate depletion of healthy men. *American Journal of Clinical Nutrition* 54, 1302S–1309S.

7. Peters, John M., et al. (1994). Processed meats and risk of childhood leukemia (California, USA). *Cancer Causes and Control* 5, 2–9.

8. Shimpo, Kan, et al. (1991). Ascorbic acid and adriamycin toxicity. *American Journal of Clinical Nutrition* 54, 1298S–1301S.

9. Packer, J. E., et al. (1979). *Nature* 278, 737–738.

10. Cheraskin, Emanuel, Ringsdorf, W. Marshall, Jr., and Sisley, Emily L. (1983). *The Vitamin C Connection* (p. 55). New York: Harper and Row.

11. Levine, Mark, et al. (1991). Ascorbic acid and in situ kinetics: A new approach to vitamin requirements. *American Journal of Clinical Nutrition* 54, 1157S.

12. Ibid.

13. Cathcart, p. 1360.

14. Pauling, Linus. (1978). Robert F. Cathcart III, MD: An orthomolecular physician. *The Linus Pauling Institute of Science and Medicine Newsletter* 1(4), 2.

15. Cathcart, p. 1373.

16. Cheraskin, p. 19.

17. Cheraskin, Emanuel. (1984). "The Vitamin C Connection." Speech delivered to the Tenth Mandala Holistic Health Conference, San Diego, September 1.

18. Hausman, Patricia. (1987). *The Right Dose: How to Take Vitamins & Minerals Safely* (p. 196). Emmaus, PA: Rodale Press.

19. Cheraskin, p. 213.

20. Hausman, p. 203.

21. Szent-Gyorgyi, A. (1977). On a substance that can make us sick (if we do not eat it!). *Executive Health* 13(9). Cited in Robbins, R. C. (1980). On Bioflavonoids. *Executive Health* 14(12), 2.

22. Hertog, Michael G. L., et al. (1993). Intake of potentially anticarcinogenic flavonoids and their determinants in adults in The Netherlands. *Nutrition and Cancer* 20(1), 21–29.

23. Piazza, Marcello, et al. (1983). Effect of (+)-cyanidanol-3 in acute HAV, HBV, and non-A, non-B viral hepatitis. *Hepatology* 3(1), 45–49.

24. Byers, Tim, et al. (1990). New directions: The diet–cancer link. *Patient Care*, November 30, 34–48.

25. Stavric, B., and Matula, T. I. (1992). Flavonoids in foods: Their significance for nutrition and health. In *Lipid Soluble Antioxidants: Biochemistry and Clinical Applications*. Cambridge, MA: Birkhauser Basel.

26. Gaby, Alan R., and Wright, Jonathan V. (1993). Nutritional factors in degenerative eye disorders: Cataract and macular degeneration. *Journal of the Advancement of Medicine* 6(1), 27–40.

27. Picq, M., et al. (1991). Effect of two flavonoid compounds on central nervous system analgesic activity. *Life Sciences* 49, 1979–1988. Cited in Hamilton, Kirk. (1992). *Clinical Pearls* (p. 375). Sacramento, CA: ITServices.

28. Middleton, E., Jr., and Drzwiecki, G. (1992). Effect of ascorbic acid and flavonoids on human basophil histamine release. *Journal of Allergy and Clinical Immunology* 89(1/Part II), 278/536. Cited in Hamilton, Kirk. (1992). *Clinical Pearls* (p. 41). Sacramento, CA: ITServices.

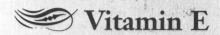 Vitamin E

According to vitamin E researcher Lester Packer of the University of California at Berkeley, "frank vitamin E deficiency is very seldom seen in humans," and yet, as Packer also points out, the vitamin is of critical importance in a number of illnesses and disorders, including heart disease, diabetes, cancer, arthritis, and cataracts and also for those exposed to strenuous exercise, air pollution, and even aging.[1] Low levels of vitamin E have also been implicated in preeclampsia (a dangerous condition of late pregnancy), sickle cell anemia, and tardive dyskinesia (a neurological disease involving involuntary movements).

Vitamin E is one of the most potent of antioxidants, protecting the fats (called *lipids*) found in cell walls and cell interiors from free radical damage (a process of destruction called *lipid peroxidation*). In fact, if you squeeze a few drops of liquid vitamin E into a new bottle of cooking oil, the vitamin will prevent rancidity and extend the life of the oil. Inside your body, the vitamin is needed in increasing amounts as the amount of polyunsaturated fatty acids, frequently consumed as corn, safflower, sunflower, and soybean cooking oils, increases in the daily diet.

One of vitamin E's special talents is an ability to stop a wildly proliferating free radical chain reaction while it is occurring. In fact, the vitamin is renown as the best lipid-soluble chain-breaking antioxidant.

In a curious twist of nature, as vitamin E is used up in the process of protecting us from free radicals, it itself forms a dangerous radical. This new form quickens the rate at which the vitamin is used up. Fortunately, vitamin C comes along as the hero in this scenario, regenerating and extending the useful life of vitamin E. Thus, if you take both vitamin E and vitamin C at the same time, less vitamin E will have the same beneficial effect of a greater amount of vitamin E taken alone.[2] Vitamin E and beta-carotene perform their own pas-de-deux, choreographed by the concentration of oxygen. Where oxygen concentration is high, such as the bloodstream, vitamin E is hard at work protecting fats circulating in the blood from spoilage. Where oxygen concentration is low, such as parts of the cell relatively far from the blood supply, beta-carotene does the job.

Which Form?

The difference between natural and synthetic forms of vitamin E has to do with their spatial arrangement. Even though molecules are too tiny to see with your eyes, they do exist in three dimensions. d-Alpha tocopherol is the name given to the form of tocopherol found in vegetable oils. dl-Alpha tocopherol refers to the product created in a laboratory. The "d" refers to the direction the molecule rotates: d is to the right (from the Latin *dextro*); l is to the left (from the Latin *laevus*). In terms of potency and levels in the blood, dl-alpha tocopherol is just as biologically active as the natural product extracted from vegetable oils.[3]

Vitamin E is actually a family of compounds, the tocopherols and tocotrienols, which are individually named after the letters of the Greek alphabet: alpha, beta, gamma, delta. The alpha form is the most biologically active in both cases.

The vitamin has numerous beneficial effects in the body, and not all of them relate to its antioxidant abilities. For example, it can prevent miscarriage and phlebitis (the inflammation of a vein, often along with a clot) and influence the production of certain hormone-like biochemicals called prostaglandins, which regulate inflammation, pain, and other important processes in the body.

Vitamin E

What are the functions of vitamin E? Vitamin E protects fats in the cell wall, in the cell interior, and in the blood from free radical destruction (lipid peroxidation). It also prevents red blood cells from clotting and sticking together; protects beta-carotene from destruction by free radicals (oxidation); works together with selenium to protect the body from free radicals; helps produce the antioxidant enzyme superoxide dismutase; helps protect the body from carcinogens, heavy metals, and industrial chemicals; reduces side effects from chemotherapeutic drugs; improves blood flow to the hands and feet; raises levels of high density lipoproteins (HDL) in the blood; reduces noncancerous lumps in the breast; helps lessen scarring internally and externally after surgery or injury; improves immune function; and reduces hot flashes.

What are the signs of deficiency? A vitamin E deficiency is marked by anemia, difficulty walking and maintaining balance, easy bleeding (capillary fragility), and by "liver spots" (accumulations of brownish colored pigmentation).

How is it absorbed into bloodstream? Vitamin E is absorbed through fats and oils in the diet.

What limits absorption? Diseases causing poor fat absorption, such as pancreatitis, deficiency of pancreatic enzymes, celiac disease, cystic fibrosis, and gall bladder disease all can limit vitamin E absorption.

What are the sources? Vitamin E is found in vegetable oils (safflower and palm are best, but vitamin E is also found in cottonseed, corn, and soybean oils) and wheat germ oil. Some vitamin E is also found in dark green leafy vegetables (kale, collard, mustard greens, chard), egg yolk, seeds, and nuts.

Who is at risk of deficiency? People who eat white rice and baked goods made with white flour, coupled with a great deal of polyunsaturated fat in their daily diet are at risk of deficiency. The higher the consumption of polyunsaturated fats and oils, the more vitamin E is needed to prevent free radical destruction of these fats and oils.

What are the signs of overdose? Toxic doses of vitamin E are characterized by fatigue, weakness, and excessive blood clotting time.

What is the Recommended Dietary Allowance (RDA)? The RDA for infants from birth to 6 months is 5 mg (1 mg = 1.49 IU of d-alpha tocopherol, so 5 mg = 7.45 IU); for those from 6 months to 1 year it is 4 mg (5.96 IU). Children from 1 to 3 years require 6 mg (8.94 IU), and those from 4 to 10 need 7 mg (10.43 IU). Males 11 and older should get 10 mg (14.9 IU), and females 11 and older need 8 mg (11.92 IU). Women who are pregnant should have 10 mg (14.9 IU); those lactating in months 1 through 6 need 12 mg (17.88 IU), while those in months 6 through 12 need 11 mg (16.39 IU).

"IU" stands for International Unit, which is the measurement of all oil-based vitamins. (If the vitamin is measured in milligrams [mg] or micrograms [mcg], it has been manufactured in a dried and powdered form, often indicated by "acetate" or "succinate" in the name on the label.)

What is the usual safe daily dose? A daily dosage of 100–800 IU is generally considered safe. Doses as high as 1,200 IU have been used for cases of poor circulation, without side effects. However, if high doses are desired, it is best to start with 100 IU and slowly build up to the desired dosage over several weeks.

Warning on supplementation: Do not take supplemental vitamin E if you are taking the blood-thinner warfarin (Coumadin®) or another anticoagulant medication.

These benefits and others are collectively called its "vitamin E activity." The difference between the vitamin's antioxidant effects and its vitamin E activity is only now becoming the focus of scientific attention.[4] Commercial manufacturers of vitamin supplements haven't yet caught up to these differences.

For example, tocotrienols have a significantly higher antioxidant effect than tocopherols. In fact, they are 10 to 20 times more potent antioxidants than are tocopherols, but what you will find in your supplements are tocopherols, particularly alpha tocopherol, because in the recent past what was emphasized was alpha tocopherol's superior vitamin E activity.

Different sources of vitamin E have differing proportions of tocopherols and tocotrienols. Among the vegetable oils, tocotrienols are mainly present in barley and palm oil. Safflower oil is the best source of alpha tocopherol (90 percent). The vitamin E in corn oil, by comparison, is only 10 percent alpha tocopherol.

Natural vitamin E as a supplement is manufactured in several forms, including d-alpha tocopherol, d-alpha tocopherol acetate, and d-alpha tocopherol succinate. Scientific studies have used all the various forms, with positive results. You, too, will most likely receive benefit from your supplement, whichever form you use. As with all antioxidants, however, don't rely exclusively on a supplement. Pay attention to food sources.

Sources

The very best sources of vitamin E are the oil-rich inner germ of wheat, barley, and other grains, and cold-pressed, unrefined palm, safflower, and other vegetable oils. The vitamin is also, in lesser amounts, in egg yolk, nuts, and legumes and in spinach, broccoli, chard, collard, mustard greens, kale, and other dark leafy green vegetables.

The more refined the oil, the more the vitamin E has been removed. Since vitamin E protects oils in your body as well as oil in bottles from oxidation damage, the more refined polyunsaturated oils you consume, the more vitamin E you need to take. Unrefined oils are advertised as such, and are often found in the health foods section of supermarkets, or in natural foods markets. They are generally of a deeper color than refined oils.

Dosage

The Recommended Dietary Allowance is 30 IU per day for adult men and women. The dosage that is best for you depends on your needs. Are you basically healthy and just want to prevent future problems with your cardiovascular system? Then 30 to 100 IU vitamin E a day is adequate.

Do you suffer from intermittent claudication? This is a sudden intense pain in the legs while walking, caused by constriction of blood vessels. Intervention trials have used anywhere from 400 to 1,600 IU of vitamin E with success. For coronary artery disease, one study used 1,200 IU per day to successfully reduce the use of nitroglycerin.

Take a look at some of the resources listed in Part III for more specific recommendations for your particular condition, and don't forget to include your health provider in the loop. He or she can offer advice, provide any needed warnings about possible drug–nutrient interactions, and possibly do a literature search for more information on the use of vitamin E for your condition.

Toxicity

Vitamin E is one of the safest vitamins, with very few side effects reported even at 800 IU per day. The major discomforts experienced by some people are fatigue and weakness. Breast pain, emotional depression, abnormal blood tests, and muscular weakness are some other reported side effects of vitamin E overdose, but are exceedingly rare.

People who are taking a blood thinning drug, such as warfarin (Coumadin®) or for any other reason have a tendency to bleed, can find high doses of vitamin E dangerous because it can extend the amount of time needed for blood to clot and can therefore lead to internal bleeding. If you are taking a blood thinner, your safest choice is to take more vitamin C and less vitamin E, since vitamin C increases the length of time vitamin E stays active in the body.

Conclusion

Vitamin E is intimately involved in the health of the cardiovascular system, skin, and nerves. It works both alone and in concert with the other antioxidants, and is an essential partner in our free radical defense forces.

Notes

1. Packer, Lester. (1992). Interaction among antioxidants in health and disease: Vitamin E and its redox cycle. *Proceedings of the Society for Experimental Biology and Medicine* 200, 271–276.
2. Personal communication with Elena Servinova, Ph.D., Department of Molecular and Cell Biology, University of California, Berkeley. May 25, 1994.
3. Baker, H., et al. (1985). Biological activities of d and dl forms of vitamin E: Comparison of plasma tocopherol levels following oral administration in humans. *Federal Proceedings* 44, 935. Cited in *The Nutrition Report* (p. 54). July 1985. San Diego: Health Media Communications.
4. Beamish, Robert E. (1993). Vitamin E—Then and now. *Canadian Journal of Cardiology* 9(1), 29–30.

≈ Selenium

Selenium is a naturally occurring element that is used in a number of industries to keep glass clear, make red lights red, and allow copy machines to conduct current when exposed to light. What interests us, however, is selenium's use as an excellent antioxidant, both on its own and particularly in concert with vitamin E. In addition, we are interested in its role as an activator of the important antioxidant enzyme called glutathione peroxidase, described in detail later.

Selenium complements the work of vitamin E. Where vitamin E serves the body as the only free-radical-trapping, fat-soluble antioxidant in the bloodstream, selenium destroys fat-soluble oxidants in the watery realm of the cell.

Selenium is found in the soil and taken up by plants. We obtain our selenium from eating these plants and the animals that eat the plants. Selenium is needed in minute amounts, measured in micrograms (mcg, millionths of a gram). However, even though so little is needed, scientists consistently find selenium levels lower than normal in patients with AIDS, cancer, arthritis, Crohn's disease, sickle cell anemia, chronic pancreatitis, multiple sclerosis, asthma, Down syndrome, and psoriasis. Sperm counts are found significantly lower in men with low selenium in their blood. Scientists also find vegetables and grains grown in certain areas naturally deficient in this important mineral.

Selenium

What are the functions of selenium? Selenium protects the liver from damage; inhibits oxidation of fats; improves assimilation of vitamin E; helps protect the body from damage due to environmental pollution, including blocking the toxic effects of heavy metals such as cadmium and mercury; helps prevent cancer; and helps prevent heart disease.

What are the signs of deficiency? Selenium deficiency is characterized by muscular pains; heart muscle degeneration; abnormal sperm; and liver, kidney, and pancreas damage.

How should you take it? Selenomethionine, the form of selenium found in plants, is better absorbed than is sodium selenite, the form usually found in supplements. For best antioxidant use, take selenium with vitamin E, as together they are essential promoters of glutathione peroxidase enzyme activity; vitamin C, in contrast, lowers selenium levels.

What are the dietary sources? The best dietary sources are fish, kidney, and liver. Another good source is selenium-enriched yeast. Other, lesser sources include cereals, poultry, nonorgan meat, and, in even lesser amounts, dairy foods. Good vegetarian sources are mushrooms, garlic, and asparagus.

Who is at risk of deficiency? People at risk for selenium

Geographic Roulette

Twenty years ago, both the United States and Canada ordered that selenium be added to poultry and swine feed, after studies revealed widely varying levels of selenium in crops grown in different areas. In feed corn, for example, the U.S. Food and Drug Administration found selenium content varying from 0.01 parts per million (ppm) to 2.03 ppm. Wheat grown in selenium-poor New Zealand can be 1,000-fold lower in selenium than wheat grown in the selenium-rich soil of South Dakota.

deficiency are those on intravenous tube feeding, those on restricted synthetic diets for various genetically induced metabolic conditions, those eating food or meat fed fodder grown in selenium-deficient areas, alcoholics, and premature babies fed a selenium-deficient infant formula.

What are the signs of overdose? The following are signs of selenium overdose: loss of hair, brittleness of fingernails, garlic odor on the breath, fatigue, and irritability.

What is the Recommended Dietary Allowance (RDA)? Infants birth to 6 months of age require 10 micrograms (mcg); those 6 months to 1 year need 15 mcg. Children from 1 to 6 years old need 20 mcg, while those from 7 to 10 should get 30 mcg. Males 11 through 14 years need 40 mcg, and those 15 to 18 require 50 mcg. Men 19 and older should get 70 mcg. Females 11 through 14 years need 45 mcg, and those 15 to 18 require 50 mcg. Women 19 and older should get 55 mcg, pregnant women need 65 mcg, and those lactating need 75 mcg.

What is the usual safe daily dose? The usual safe dose ranges from 50 to 200 mcg.

Warning on supplementation: Selenium can be toxic at 1,000 mcg (1 mg) per day.

When Dr. Raymond J. Shamberger, formerly of the Cleveland Clinic, studied the geographic distribution of human cancer and heart disease, he found a direct parallel to selenium levels in the soil. The lowest cancer rate was in Rapid City, South Dakota, which measured highest for selenium in the population's blood. Lima, Ohio, residents had the lowest levels of selenium in their blood, and the highest cancer rate. A similar pattern emerged for heart disease, with people living in selenium-poor states three times more likely to die from heart disease than those living in selenium-rich areas.

Where do you live? In the United States, North and South Dakota have the highest levels of selenium. Alabama, Arizona, Colorado, Kansas, Louisiana, Nebraska, Oklahoma, Texas, and Utah have medium levels. Selenium-poor states include Connecticut, Delaware, Illinois, Indiana, Massachusetts, New York, Ohio, Oregon, Pennsylvania, and Rhode Island. The District of Columbia is selenium deficient as are parts of Florida, Maine, Michigan, New Hampshire, Vermont, and Washington.

If you live in a selenium-poor area and are consuming locally grown food, supplementation may be necessary to maintain the recommended minimum daily intake of from 50 to 200 mcg.

Form Is Important

The kind of selenium found in food is called selenomethionine, an organic form of the mineral. The form of selenium sometimes found in nutritional supplements is called sodium selenite, which is inorganic and less easily absorbed. Thus, it is likely that when you obtain your selenium from the food you eat, more of it goes into your tissues than when you take a similar amount in supplement form.[1]

Getting Enough

If an institutionalized loved one is on tube feeding (called TPN for total parenteral nutrition), ask questions about the formula being used. A study in Chicago published in the *American Journal of Clinical Nutrition* in 1987 found patients on TPN with serum selenium levels below normal. The patients also had low levels of glutathione peroxidase, a selenium-dependent antioxidant enzyme.[2] The researchers concluded that intravenous nutrition formulas should contain more than 100 mcg of selenium to keep patients at normal levels of this important anti-cancer, anti-heart-disease antioxidant.

Preterm infants fed infant formula instead of breast milk are another group at risk of selenium deficiency. A joint study by the University of Guelph and the Neonatal Intensive Care Unit at

McMaster Medical Center in Ontario, Canada, found commercial infant formulas that did not offer low birthweight premature infants adequate amounts of selenium (10–15 mcg).[3]

No one seems to know what causes dandruff, a scaling of the scalp. A major brand of anti-dandruff shampoo contains 1 percent selenium sulfide, and even incorporates the "sel" of selenium into its name. Could dandruff be a sign of selenium deficiency?

Toxicity

More than most other trace minerals, selenium has quite a narrow margin between a too small and a too great dosage. Back in the 1930s, scientists were more worried about selenium excess than deficiency. Animals grazing on selenium-excessive soil lost their appetite and their hair, stopped growing, became emaciated, and moved stiffly. Ranchers in these areas would find their horses and cattle suffering from the "blind staggers," a condition that left the animals awkwardly staggering across the field as though they could not see or coordinate their movements.

In 1987, the public was shocked by photos of hundreds of migratory birds deformed or killed at a wildlife refuge in the western San Joaquin Valley of California. The cause was a mystery until scientists found elevated selenium levels in the ponds at the refuge due to an accumulation of agricultural wastewater there.

Humans who are poisoned from too much selenium will also lose their hair, will have brittle fingernails and a garlic odor on their breath, and will suffer from fatigue and irritability.

Conclusion

Selenium is an important part of an antioxidant defense formula. It prevents heavy metal toxicity and stimulates the anti-cancer power of glutathione peroxidase. The mineral plays a key role in maintaining a strong immune system and in preventing cancer, heart disease, arthritis, and degenerative changes in your liver, kidneys, and pancreas. It may play an unrecognized role in male infertility and in the minor but aggravating condition known as dandruff.

Notes

1. Whanger, P. (1986). Some comparative aspects of selenite and selenomethionine metabolism. *Journal of the American College of Toxicology* 5, 101–110.

2. Feller, A., et al. (1987). Subnormal concentrations of serum selenium and plasma carnitine in chronically tube-fed patients. *American Journal of Clinical Nutrition* 45, 476–483.

3. Friel, J., et al. (1985). Selenium and chromium intakes of very low birthweight pre-term and normal birthweight full-term infants during the first twelve months. *Nutrition Research* 5, 1175–1184.

Coenzyme Q10

Inside each body cell is a power plant called a mitochondrion. Inside this cellular power plant a number of sequenced steps occur to produce the energy that keeps us alive and moving. Whenever several steps are necessary to produce an end product, the body usually speeds up the process using a special protein called an enzyme. Sometimes two or more substances must combine to produce one enzyme. These substances are called *coenzymes*, and in mitochondria one of the most important coenzymes keeps the power plant fires stoked and burning. Its name is coenzyme Q10 (CoQ10), and in addition to facilitating the production of energy, coenzyme Q10 is a powerful antioxidant and free radical scavenger.

CoQ10 is found in abundance in the heart, which needs a constant and assured source of energy to keep pumping day and night for many decades. CoQ10 is also found in the fat of cell membranes. It isn't coincidental that this is the same neighborhood where vitamin E resides. Just as all good governments contain a check and balance of power, so all successful biological systems provide for a check and balance of potentially harmful substances. In certain specific conditions, vitamin E is altered to become a radical (a fragment of its former self) and instead of protecting low density lipoproteins (a blood fat) from oxidation, the vitamin E itself initiates the oxidation. In these cases, along comes CoQ10, in addition to vitamin C, to protect the LDL cholesterol from oxidation by the vitamin E radical. Since oxidized LDL damages arteries, CoQ10 protects the body from cardiovascular disease.[1] More on this supplement for cardiovascular health is found on pages 148–149.

People with cancer can benefit from CoQ10's ability to diminish heart problems. Adriamycin and other chemotherapeutic drugs are hard on the heart. Studies of human patients as well as of animals have found a remarkable elimination of cardiovascular side effects when cancer patients take CoQ10 along with their medication.[2]

With CoQ10, it is possible people with cancer will handle their tumors before needing chemotherapy. Dr. Karl Folkers, of the Institute for Biomedical Research at University of Texas at Austin, recently reported that CoQ10, along with vitamins and minerals, caused breast tumors to regress and to disappear when the daily CoQ10 dosage was increased to 300 mg.[3]

Dr. Denham Harman of Omaha, Nebraska, was a pioneer in linking free radicals to the process of aging. Recently, Harman explained a hypothesis linking Alzheimer's disease to free-radical-initiated mutation of DNA. Harman's scenario has this DNA damage occurring early in life, even during fetal development, though the consequences are not evident until the person is middle aged or older. The consequences include an accumulation of hydrogen peroxide and hydroxyl radical, both potent oxidants that Harman believes have a role in the development of Alzheimer's disease in susceptible individuals. Harman sees coenzyme Q10 and vitamin sources of antioxidants as temporarily able to improve mental function even in cases of Alzheimer's.[4]

A Japanese study evaluated 21 patients with chronic obstructive lung disease and idiopathic pulmonary fibrosis at rest and after exercise, both before and after 8 weeks of taking 90 mg of CoQ10.[5] At the study's end, those taking the enzyme had greater oxygen uptake measured at rest, their heart rate had significantly decreased, and their performance increased during exercise. The researchers concluded that CoQ10 has favorable effects on muscular energy metabolism.

Frustrated dentists and patients with the "no hope" diagnosis of gum disease have found that complete relief from the problem is possible after CoQ10 therapy.[6] Read more about periodontal disease treatment with CoQ10 on pages 164–165.

Dosage and Toxicity

The usual dose of CoQ10 used in clinical trials is 30–100 mg daily. In studies lasting up to 6 years, no toxicity has been found.

Conclusion

Coenzyme Q10 is an excellent addition to your self-help pharmacy if you are suffering from some abnormality of your cardiovascular system or lung function or if you are working to heal from cancer or periodontitis. It is a potent energy source, and a powerful antioxidant.

Notes

1. Stocker, R. (1992). Dietary supplementation with coenzyme Q10 results in increased levels of ubiquinol-10 within circulating lipoproteins and increased resistance of human low-density lipoprotein to the initiation of lipid peroxidation. *Biochimica et Biophysica ACTA* 1126, 247–254.

2. Bliznakov, Emile G., and Hunt, Gerald L. (1987). *The Miracle Nutrient: Coenzyme Q10* (pp. 135–139). New York: Bantam.

3. Folkers, Karl, et al. (1994). Partial and complete regression of breast cancer in patients in relation to dosage of coenzyme Q10. *Biochemical and Biophysical Research Communications* 199(3), 1504–1508.

4. Harman, Denham, (1993). Free radical theory of ageing: A hypothesis on pathogenesis of senile dementia of the Alzheimer's type. Age 16, 23–30. Cited in Hamilton, Kirk. (1993). *Clinical Pearls* (p. 17). Sacramento, CA: ITServices.

5. Fujimoto, S. (1993). Effects of coenzyme Q10 administration on pulmonary function and exercise performance in patients with chronic lung disease. *Clinical Investigator* 71, S162–S166. Cited in Hamilton, Kirk. (1993). *Clinical Pearls* (p. 264). Sacramento, CA: ITServices.

6. Bliznakov, pp. 140–149.

⤳ Cysteine

Cysteine is an amino acid. It joins with other amino acids to form proteins. However, cysteine's most remarkable ability may be the ease with which it can detoxify harmful chemicals and heavy metals. It has been used to prevent poisoning and to treat a wide variety of conditions ranging from bronchitis to psychosis.

Why It Works

What gives cysteine its power is the sulfur-containing thiol group in its chemical composition. Sulfur has been used to treat medical conditions for thousands of years, and is found in sulfur-rich hot springs, in garlic and onions, and in pharmaceuticals such as merthiolate, an antibacterial product that not so long ago was in everyone's first aid kit.

Cysteine's thiol group serves as a handy reducing agent, which means it prevents the destruction of healthy tissues by an act of self-sacrifice. The thiol group in cysteine allows itself to be oxidized first, protecting and preserving the integrity of healthy tissues around it.

Cysteine is a powerful scavenger of hydrogen peroxide, which is a damaging form of oxygen that is released during any kind of inflammation.

Glutathione is a biochemical created by the body to protect us against free radical damage. The amount of glutathione in the blood changes according to how much cysteine is in the diet:

Whenever the liver finds enough cysteine in the blood, it produces more glutathione. And, we definitely want as much glutathione as we can get! Glutathione has been called "the toxic waste neutralizer of the body"[1] by Eric Braverman and Carl Pfeiffer in their book *The Healing Nutrients: Facts, Findings, and New Research on Amino Acids.* When glutathione is exhausted in the process of protecting us from free radicals, cysteine helps it recover and continue its work.

N-acetylcysteine (NAC), a cysteine derivative, has proved extremely useful as an intravenous antidote to acetaminophen poisoning. Such poisoning causes liver damage and is especially common when this drug is taken for long periods of time with alcohol. Liver damage is also possible due to allergic reactions to the drug, which include fever-and pain-reducers such as Tylenol and Anacin.

A number of reports find NAC useful in preventing side effects from powerful drugs and radiation treatments used to fight cancer.

Other uses for cysteine include regrowing hair (among women) and reducing heavy metal toxicity when lead, copper, or cobalt poisoning has occurred.

Although one randomized, double-blind, placebo-controlled study did not prove N-acetylcysteine useful for adult respiratory distress syndrome,[2] in other instances it has been prescribed specifically for respiratory conditions because it is able to liquify mucus that has thickened in the lungs. N-acetylcysteine has been used for adult respiratory distress syndrome, as well as Acquired Immune Deficiency Syndrome (AIDS), asthma, emphysema, cystic fibrosis, lung abscess, chronic obstructive pulmonary disease, and chronic bronchitis. Chronic bronchitis, for example, has responded to morning and evening dosages of 200 mg of NAC.

Cysteine versus NAC

Much of the research on cysteine has been with NAC, since only the derivative, a laboratory-created substance, can be patented. However, some NAC converts back into cysteine in the body, and the research proving NAC's usefulness can be applied to cysteine, as well.[3]

There are several benefits of cysteine over NAC. One is, it's cheaper. Another is its smell and taste are much more acceptable than NAC's. Braverman and Pfeiffer note that even pregnant women can take up to 10 grams of NAC a day, but may not want to due to the chemical's nauseating smell and taste. Happily, cysteine doesn't have this problem.

In addition, say the researchers, large intravenous doses of NAC can cause hyperactivity, loss of balance, and—with extremely high doses—convulsions can occur. None of these side effects are associated with cysteine.

Food Sources of Cysteine

You can find cysteine in garlic, onions, asparagus, red peppers, meat, cabbage, brussels sprouts, broccoli, cauliflower, mustard, and horseradish. When taken in supplemental form, amino acids like cysteine need to be consumed on an empty stomach (except for other "helper" supplements), or they are used by the body as food and not as a therapeutic agent.

Nutrient Helpers

Selenium

Since cysteine supplementation increases production of glutathione peroxidase, the body's great free radical scavenger, and since the mineral selenium is an important part of the glutathione compound, it is useful to take selenium along with cysteine.

Vitamin C

Cysteine and vitamin C make a powerful pair when they fight oxidants together. Both are strong anti-toxins, protecting the body from environmental pollutants such as pesticides, herbicides, heavy metals, hydrocarbons (as in smog), pharmaceutical drugs, bacteria, and chemicals.

Dosage

When taking cysteine along with its nutrient helpers, the proper dosage of cysteine is 500 mg once a day, along with 200 mcg of selenium and 1,000 mg of vitamin C.

Conclusion

Cysteine, one of the least known of the antioxidants, is best taken on an empty stomach along with selenium and vitamin C to help in cases of respiratory ailments, environmental pollution, and drug overdoses, particularly acetaminophen. A pharmaceutical derivative of cysteine, called N-acetylcysteine or NAC, has also proved useful.

Notes

1. Braverman, Eric R., and Pfeiffer, Carl C. (1987). *The Healing Nutrients Within: Facts, Findings and New Research on Amino Acids* (p. 90). New Canaan, CT: Keats Publishing.
2. Jepsen, S., et al. (1992). Antioxidant treatment with N-acetylcysteine during adult respiratory distress syndrome: A prospective, randomized, placebo-controlled study. *Critical Care Medicine* 20(7), 918[en]923.
3. Braverman, p. 94.

≫ Melatonin

Melatonin is a hormone released from the pineal gland. A simple derivative of the amino acid tryptophan and the neurotransmitter serotonin, melatonin appears in the blood in a recurring, daily cycle, with nighttime levels as much as ten times greater than those measured during the day. It is an efficient, powerful free radical scavenger, so effective in removing toxic hydroxyl molecules from circulation in the bloodstream[1] that it has been called "the most potent free radical scavenger to date."[2]

Like much of nutritional medicine, there are contradictions in the use of this natural substance. Studies link adequate melatonin with retarding the process of aging,[3] and too little melatonin with increased risk of prostate and breast cancer. [4] In fact, the increase of melatonin at night is associated with antitumor activity, yet it is believed that the relief of depression enjoyed by people with Seasonal Affective Disorder (depression caused by a lack of bright sunshine) is due to the suppression of melatonin during the daylight hours.[5]

Jet-lagged travelers, shift workers, the blind, and the elderly have benefitted from melatonin's unique ability to provide short-term relief from insomnia and to reset their biological clocks.[6]

Dosage

Doses ranging from as little as 5 mg to as much as 5 grams have been used by various people with sleep disturbances. Earl Mindell, pharmacist and author (*The Vitamin Bible*), recommends taking 3–6 mg 1½ hours before you wish to sleep.[7]

Notes

1. Poeggeler, B., et al. (1993). Melatonin, hydroxyl radical-mediated oxidative damage, and ageing: A hypothesis. *Journal of Pineal Research* 14, 151-168. Cited in Hamilton, Kirk. (1993). *Clinical Pearls* (p. 3). Sacramento, CA: ITServices.

2. Reiter, Russel J., et al. (1993). Antioxidant capacity of melatonin: A novel action not requiring a receptor. *Neuroendocrinology Letter* 15(1,2), 103-116. Cited in Hamilton (1993), p. 302.

3. Sardi, Bill. (1992). Documented health benefits of light. *Townsend Letter for Doctors*, November, pp. 950-955. Cited in Hamilton, Kirk. (1992). Clinical Pearls (p. 255). Sacramento, CA: ITServices. *See also Poeggeler*, p. 3.

4. Sardi, p. 3.

5. Stevens, R. G., and Savitz, David. (1992). Are electromagnetic fields and cancer an issue worthy of study? Cancer 69(2), 603–605. Cited in Hamilton (1992), p. 123. *See also* Stevens, Richard G., et al. (1992). Electric power, pineal function and the risk of breast cancer. FASEB Journal, February, 6, 853-860. Cited in Hamilton (1992). p. 108.

6. Short, R. V. (1993). Melatonin: Hormone of darkness [editorial]. *British Medical Journal* 307(6910), 952-953.

7. Mindell, Earl. (1994). Stay healthy: A dosage update on melatonin. *Let's Live*, July, p. 10.

Bilberry

British Royal Air Force pilots had a sweet secret during World War II: bilberry jam. They claimed the jam improved their night vision and ability to hit targets during bombing raids. Experiments show the pilots weren't so far off their mark!

Bilberry (*Vaccinium myrtillus*) is a form of European blueberry. It grows in the northern United States and Canada in sandy soil, as well as in the meadows of northern Europe. While the North American blueberry has little medicinal power, the bilberry is rich with health benefits. Its active ingredients are flavonoids called *anthocyanosides (an-tho-sigh-an-o-sides)*.

Thanks to its anthocyanosides, the bilberry can help conditions of the eyes, connective tissue, and blood vessels.[1] For example, bilberry:

- improves how well you can see in the daytime as well as at night
- helps your eyes adapt to darkness
- helps prevent and treat cataracts, glaucoma, retinitis pigmentosa, and macular degeneration
- strengthens capillaries to prevent bleeding under the surface of the skin; to prevent and treat varicose veins, hemorrhoids, edema (water retention), and skin ulcers; and to prevent stroke

- helps protect the body's collagen, the protein substance that gives tendons, ligaments, cartilage, and skin its tensile strength and shape
- aids in keeping red blood cells from clumping together, protecting the body from blood clots that might lead to heart attacks
- helps relax smooth muscle, which is the kind of muscle lining the uterus; it thereby helps relieve menstrual cramps
- helps keep blood sugar at an even level in cases of diabetes
- helps reduce tissue destruction and uric acid levels in cases of gout

For all its powers, bilberry is amazingly safe. Anthocyanoside extracts have been taken even by pregnant women in research projects with no toxic effects. Excessive levels are excreted in the urine.

In Europe, standardized extract of bilberry is one of the most purchased herbal remedies for problems related to vision and, particularly, to the blood supply to the eyes. The herb strengthens the capillaries that deliver nutrient-rich blood to the various parts of the eye, including the muscles and nerves that serve the eyeball. By strengthening the walls of the capillaries, bilberry decreases the leakage through the capillaries of blood and substances in the blood that would damage surrounding tissues.

If there is inflammation in the eye, bilberry protects the collagen from breaking down under attack by enzymes released by the inflammatory process. Bilberry is also a fine free radical scavenger, protecting the collagen and other surfaces in the eye from damage by free radical chain reactions.

Capillary Hero: Hemorrhoids, Varicose Veins, Stroke, Bleeding Gums

All flavonoids have the ability to strengthen capillary walls. This makes them a find remedy for vascular disorders of many kinds, not only in the eye. Bruising, after all, is simply damage to capillary walls beneath the skin due to trauma, allowing blood to flow into surrounding tissues. Veins have tiny muscles around them and tiny valves within them that usually keep blood flowing in one direction: toward the heart. If blood vessel walls are weak, the blood pushes against the valve, opens it backwards, and allows the backflow to pool into painful enlarged veins. When this happens in the rectum we call it hemorrhoids. When it happens on the thighs, we call it varicose veins. Bleeding gums are a result of weak capillaries in the mouth. When capillary walls are weak in the brain, a hemorrhage can be deadly or debilitating. Bilberry seems able to reduce the inflammation that accompanies all the above vascular conditions.

In cases of edema, fluids that should stay inside the blood vessels are released into surrounding tissues. Bilberry extract in a dose of 160–320 mg per day was given to pregnant women in one 1978 study, and it was found capable of strengthening capillaries sufficiently to relieve the pooling of fluids in ankles and feet and to relieve hemorrhoids after 1 month of supplementation.[2]

Capillary Hero: Blood–Brain Barrier

Capillary walls can also be weak without actually allowing a break in their surface. They can stop working effectively as a vigilant gatekeeper. Usually, the walls have an intelligence about what to let pass through them, especially in the brain. This protects our mental functioning from damage by some drugs and chemicals. This is called the *blood–brain barrier*. Sometimes, however, capillary walls lose their ability to regulate what comes in and goes out, particularly when attacked by free radicals. Then, toxins that usually are protected from entering the brain can pass through and affect the way we think and feel. Thanks to bilberry's abilities as a free radical scavenger, it can maintain our capillaries as effective gatekeepers.[3]

Digestive Problems

Another area of the body where bilberry comes to the rescue is in stomach and intestinal problems. Bilberry causes the stomach to secrete extra mucus, protecting the lining from ulcers.

Because the berries are astringent, they have been used for diarrhea for centuries.

Dosage

You will want to purchase a brand of bilberry that claims a guaranteed anthocyanoside potency of 25 percent, a potency which conforms to that used in European research on the berry.

How much of the extract you need depends on the seriousness of your condition. Remember, taking any herb is not the same as popping an aspirin. You may have to wait for some weeks before the extract creates a noticeable difference in your vision, or an improvement in your condition. So, don't give up too soon! You don't have to be a fighter pilot to enjoy the benefit of bilberries. But, you do have to give them time to work. For prevention of eye conditions, 60–180 mg per day is recommended; to treat chronic conditions, use 300 mg per day.

Notes

1. Schechter, Steven R. (1994). Herbs for life—Bilberry extract: Nature's circulatory, visionary aid. *Let's Live*, March, 69–70.
2. Talbert, Lee, and Pauly, Michelle M. (1991). *Bilberry, An Extraordinary Vision Enhancer* (p. 9). American Institute of Health and Nutrition.
3. Murray, Michael (ed.). (1990). Vaccinium myrtillus: Collagen stabilizer. *Phyto-Pharmica Review* 3(4), 2.

~~~ Garlic

Garlic, called "Russian penicillin" during World War II, is said to be the safety net against heart disease for people around the Mediterranean. It is actually true that heart disease is quite low in Spain and Italy compared to Scotland, where vegetables are not that nation's favorite food.

The pungent bulb has impressive talents. It reduces LDL, the bad-for-you form of cholesterol; increases HDL, the good form of cholesterol; reduces blood pressure; improves blood flow to the arms and legs; and most important for our purposes, also prevents fats other than LDL cholesterol from being oxidized or from infiltrating the blood vessel wall. One speaker at the 4th International Congress on Phytotherapy, held in Munich in 1992, noted that no other antioxidant could claim as many triumphant benefits to cardiovascular health as garlic![1]

In fact, garlic has a several-thousand-year-old reputation as a potent healing agent for a wide range of conditions. Many dozens of scientific studies verify that the herb's reputation is well earned. For example, in addition to being an apparent preventive of heart attacks and strokes, garlic also seems to protect against cancer formation.[2] It kills bacteria, fungus, yeasts, viruses, and parasites.[3] It binds to and removes lead and mercury from the body.[4] And it has proven useful for lung conditions such as colds, asthma, bronchitis—even tuberculosis.[5]

66

Controversy rages over the benefits of raw garlic cloves versus the deodorized extracts in tablet or capsule form that are sold in health-food stores. According to Eric Block, professor of chemistry at State University of New York at Albany, "different garlic preparations can have different potential health benefits."[6] Raw garlic, for example, is a better antibiotic than deodorized garlic, because it retains its smelly allicin content (allicin is formed as soon as a garlic clove is crushed). Yet, deodorized garlic can control free radicals, improve immune function, prevent tumors, and lower cholesterol. Block, who discovered a garlic compound he named *ajoene*, an excellent blood-thinner, points out that onions, leeks, scallions, and chives also contain similar compounds to garlic.

Dosage

If you work at home and can avoid the social consequences of garlic breath and perspiration, consume 2–3 raw garlic cloves a day and cook garlic regularly in your everyday meals. If your daily life includes regular contact with people, take raw garlic whenever possible, and as a daily preventive supplement take 2–3 tablets or capsules of a deodorized brand 3 times a day. Six tablets of deodorized extract equal approximately one clove of fresh garlic.

Notes

1. Fogarty, M. (1993). Garlic's potential role in reducing heart disease. *British Journal of Clinical Practice* 47(2), 64–65. Cited in Hamilton, Kirk. (1993). *Clinical Pearls* (p. 92). Sacramento, CA: ITServices.
2. Long, Patricia. (1988). Garlic: It gets in your blood. *Hippocrates*, January–February, p. 18.
3. Sandhu, D. K., et al. (1980). Sensitivity of yeasts isolated from cases of vaginitis to aqueous extracts of garlic. *Mykosen* 23(12), 691.
4. Block, Eric. Personal communication, April 17, 1991.
5. Carper, Jean. *The Food Pharmacy* (pp. 199 and 203). New York: Bantam.
6. Block, Eric. Personal communication, April 17, 1991.

❧ Ginkgo Biloba

The first ginkgo tree in America was planted in Philadelphia some 200 years ago. Ginkgos also grace the streets in Washington, D.C., New York, Sacramento, and many other downtowns in between. I wonder if any city employees who chose the ornamental tree know that an extract of its leaves is currently one of the most frequently prescribed medicines in France and Germany.

Ginkgo trees have actually been on earth over 200 million years, predating the dinosaurs! The tree is native to China but the tree's name is derived from the Japanese word *ginkyo* and, because the leaves have two lobes, its botanical name became Ginkgo biloba. In the fall the trees wear yellowing leaves rich with flavonoids (*flavo* means yellow). These flavonoids provide the herb's antioxidant power.

In recent years, the herb's most powerful constituents have been synthesized by Harvard researchers. Eventually, with the usual economic imperative, a laboratory version of individual components of the extract will most likely be marketed, and most likely it will be by prescription. When that happens, it will be good to recall that scientists from the Department of Epidemiology, University of Limburg, The Netherlands, found so many active ingredients in ginkgo extract, and so many sites in the body where the compounds are active, they concluded the constituents probably act synergistically (the combination is more powerful than ordinarily expected).[1] This means something worthwhile may be lost if only one constituent is pulled out and used medicinally.

Herbal Antioxidant

Dr. Donald Brown, a naturopathic physician and faculty member at Bastyr University in Seattle, points out that the human brain has a higher proportion of unsaturated fats among brain cells than anywhere else in the body.[2] It is, therefore, no wonder that ginkgo, which protects those fats from free radical destruction (lipid peroxidation), has proven itself effective in improving memory, reducing the effects of head injury, improving concentration, accelerating learning, increasing blood flow and oxygenation of tissues throughout the body, improving the transmission of nerve signals, and generally improving brain function. Ginkgo also helps relieve migraine headaches. When ginkgo extract was given to patients suffering migraines in an open trial back in 1975, there was an improvement or a near-total cure in 80 percent of sufferers.[3]

The herb has also been used with patients suffering from Alzheimer's disease,[4] but you don't have to be senile to benefit from ginkgo. In a double-blind study of elderly patients who did not have Alzheimer's, ginkgo improved performance on tests of mental acuity and memory, and those patients with the most deteriorated initial condition improved the most.

Even healthy young minds work better after consuming ginkgo. In 1988, Hindmarch reported his study of standardized ginkgo extract capsules on the short-term memory of volunteers ages 25 to 40. He used a double-blind crossover trial, and found just 1 hour after participants consumed one 600-mg dose of ginkgo, their short-term memory significantly improved. This improvement was not apparent at doses of 120 or 240 mg.[5]

Ginkgo's flavonoid glycosides are particularly adept at improving circulation and at strengthening the walls of our tiniest blood vessels, the capillaries. Since this improves blood flow to the brain, why not other parts further south? When 60 men who

were unable to maintain an erection and who had not responded
to the usual drug therapy (papaverine injections) were given 60
mg of ginkgo per day, by 6 months into the study 50 percent of
them could maintain erections.[6]

Organ Transplants

The problem with organ transplants, once a proper donor organ
has been found, is preventing the body from rejecting the new
organ. The ginkgolides in ginkgo biloba are able to interfere with
this rejection cycle by halting the work of a certain chemical called
platelet activating factor (PAF). With rats, at least, ginkgo pro-
longs the survival time of those with grafted hearts. Research continues with great hopes that ginkgo may serve as an alternative to
the usual immunosuppressive drug used for transplants—
cyclosporin, which has many dangerous and undesirable side
effects.

Toxicity

Ginkgo is quite safe. In very rare cases, mild gastrointestinal complaints, headache, and allergic skin reactions have been reported,[7]
which are quickly relieved by lowering the amount of herb consumed. In addition, there are no drug interactions with Ginkgo
biloba.

   According to Kleijnen and Knipschild of the University of
Limburg, The Netherlands, "no serious side effects have been
noted in any trial and, if present, side effects were no different
from those in patients treated with placebo."[8]

Dosage

It was a German scientist, Dr. Willmar Schwabe of Schwabe
GmbH, who created a standardized (24 percent ginkgo flavone
glycoside and 6 percent terpenoid) concentrated extract of the
leaves. Schwabe's extract is known in Europe generically as EGb

761 and is marketed by prescription only. In America, we're luckier. Numerous companies sell Ginkgo biloba under their own brand in natural food markets and by mail order. Please note, however, that Schwabe's standardization (24 percent) is still the desired potency, whatever the brand.

In general, it's best for the body and for the purse to take the lowest possible dose of any supplement that will provide you the results you desire. Just be sure you give any herb, ginkgo included, time to prove its worth.

Begin with 180 mg Ginkgo biloba per day. After 4 weeks, if you don't feel a difference, take 300 mg per day. After another month, if still no results, take 600 mg per day. If you suffer gastrointestinal distress or headache from this dose, cut back until a comfortable dose is found.

Notes

1. Kleijnen, Jos, and Knipschild, Paul. (1992). Ginkgo biloba. *The Lancet* 340, 1136–1139.
2. Brown, Donald J. (1992). Ginkgo biloba—Old and new: Part I. *Let's Live*, April, 46–49.
3. Dalet, R. (1975). Essai du Tanakan dans les Cephalees et les Migraines. *Extr. vie Med.* 35, 2971–2973. Cited in Murray, Frank. (1993). *Ginkgo Biloba* (p.21). New Canaan, CT: Keats.
4. Murray, Michael T. (1990). Ginkgo biloba: "The living fossil," Part 2. *Phyto-Pharmica Review* 3(4), 1.
5. Hindmarch, I. (1988). Activity of Ginkgo biloba extract on short-term memory. In Fünfgeld, E. W. (ed.), Rökan (Ginkgo biloba), *Recent Results in Pharmacology and Clini.* Berlin: Springer-Verlag. Cited in Foster, Steven. (1990). Ginkgo. Austin, TX: American Botanical Council, Botanical Series 304.
6. Murray, pp. 3–4.
7. Kleijnen, pp. 1136–1139.
8. Kleignen, p. 1138.

~~~ Tea

Next to water, tea is the most consumed beverage in the world; yet even within any one population, tea consumption can vary from 0 to over 20 cups a day. For those of you who have conscientiously chosen the more exotic herbal tea blends over ordinary caffeine-containing green and black varieties, you may be able to switch back as you please, without guilt. In fact, there appears to be significant health benefits to green and black tea. They both contain polyphenols, which are somewhat similar to bioflavonoids and have antioxidant effects. These teas also contain a small quantity of carotenoids (including beta-carotene), which influence the tea's aroma.[1] Both green and black tea prevent the formation of nitrosamines in the stomach when nitrate-containing foods are consumed. In this way they help prevent cancer.[2]

The most important group among the antioxidant components of tea are called catechins. They control rancidity in fats and oils by halting free radical peroxide activity. Green tea, particularly, is a better free radical scavenger than even vitamin C or vitamin E when it comes to certain oxygen radicals, though not with all of them. At an international symposium on the health effects of tea, held in March 1991 at the American Health Foundation in New York, researchers reported lowered risk of heart disease and cancer in populations regularly consuming green tea (in Asia) or black tea (in parts of Europe and the United States).[3]

Green tea is manufactured from fresh leaves which are

72

crushed and heated soon after harvesting. The leaves maintain their green color and retain more polyphenols than do leaves in black tea. Black tea is allowed to lie for hours after being crushed, causing the leaves to darken. Nevertheless, the black teas still contain polyphenols that are thought at least as potent in free radical control as green teas.

Frequently, the term "tannins" is used to identify the catechins in general and the black tea's catechin oxidation products, but this is incorrect, as there is no tannic acid (used as a "tanning" agent in the manufacture of leather) in tea.[4]

In some nutritionally compromised populations drinking extremely hot tea, esophageal cancer increases. Tea has been associated with increased cancer in the Caribbean, Argentina, Brazil, Italy, parts of Japan, and in Kazakhstan. This contradiction is not unique in nature (oxygen itself is either a life giver or a danger under differing conditions); whether the tea is a danger or a lifesaver depends on the nutrition status of the individual, the level of metals in the body, and other factors. In general, for the population reading this book, tea can serve as a beneficial addition to the daily diet, as it has in Japan, where heavy smoking has not lead to the same level of lung cancer as it has in America. Some researchers suspect it's the Japanese habit of drinking green tea that is at least partly responsible.[5]

Toxicity

Tea contains about 3 percent caffeine and 0.1 and 0.02 percent, respectively, of theobromine and theophylline, which are in a family of compounds called methylxanthines. These constituents have biological effects that may not be desirable.

Pregnant women, for example, need to be careful of overenthusiastic consumption of tea. Women drinking 8½ cups of tea a day were nearly three times more likely to have slower growing fetuses and to deliver low birthweight babies in one research study.[6] In addition, there is accumulating evidence of an effect of caffeine on fertility and spontaneous miscarriage.[7]

The quantity of caffeine in tea is low, so that the caffeine content of 20 cups of tea is less than 1 gram of caffeine. However, it is there, and an enthusiastic consumption of tea might affect some sensitive individuals.

People with kidney disease or a tendency to create kidney stones (because these patients need more water in their diet),[8] women having difficulty getting pregnant or with a history of miscarriage, and women whose benign breast lumps can be eliminated by eliminating coffee and tea from their diet should avoid drinking large quantities of tea.

Dosage

According to Dr. John H. Weisburger, a pioneering tea researcher at the American Health Foundation, tea can be considered a vegetable extract. "The USDA's new food pyramid recommends five to nine servings of fruit and vegetables per day, and five cups of tea is equivalent to two of those vegetables," says Weisburger. So consider including tea as a regular part of your healthy diet for preventing cancer and heart disease.

Notes

1. Graham, Harold N. (1992). Green tea composition, consumption, and polyphenol chemistry. *Preventive Medicine* 21(3), 334–350.
2. Stich, Hans F. (1992). Teas and tea components as inhibitors of carcinogen formation in model systems and man. *Preventive Medicine* 21(3), 381–382.
3. Weisburger, John H. (1992). Physiological and pharmacological effects of *Camellia sinensis* (tea): First international symposium. *Preventive Medicine* 21(3), 329–391.
4. Graham, p. 347.
5. Carey, Benedict. (1994). Food—America's coolest new trend. *Health*, July–August, 32.
6. Dlugosz, Larry, and Brachen, Michael B. (1992). Reproductive effects of caffeine: A review and theoretical analysis. *Epidemiologic Reviews* 14, 83–100. Cited in Hamilton, Kirk. (1993). *Clinical Pearls* (p. 157). Sacramento, CA: ITServices.

7. Srisuphan, W., and Bracken, M. (1986). Caffeine consumption during pregnancy and association with late spontaneous abortion. *American Journal of Obstetrics and Gynecology* 154, 14. Cited in Reuben, Carolyn. (1992). *The Healthy Baby Book: A Parent's Guide to Preventing Birth Defects and Other Long-Term Medical Problems Before, During, and After Pregnancy* (p. 77). New York: Jeremy Tarcher.

8. Hughes, Janey, and Norman, Richard W. (1992). Diet and calcium stones. *Canadian Medical Association Journal* 146(2), 137–143. Cited in Hamilton, p. 305.

9. Weisburger, John H. Personal communication, August 24, 1994.

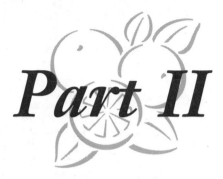

Part II

Preventing and Healing
Disease with Antioxidants

Much has been written in the medical literature and the popular press about aging, cancer, and heart disease. Part II provides lengthy chapters on each of these conditions. However, there are many other conditions that medical research has indicated are prevented, relieved, or eliminated with proper antioxidant therapy. You'll find quite a variety described here, from acne to varicose veins, and if you don't find a condition you currently have, you can proceed to Part III, where you will learn how to gather further health information for yourself.

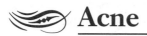 Acne

Acne is basically pimples on the face, neck, shoulders, and upper back, which can become infected and, when chronic, may cause severe scarring. Acne is probably caused by a combination of factors, though an exact cause is still unknown. Some experts suggest nutritional deficiencies and food allergies. It could be that male sex hormones influence the oil glands in affected areas, predisposing them to infection by the bacteria that live near hair follicles, but a more likely explanation is a combination of all the above, on top of a low fiber, high fat, high sugar, and refined carbohydrate Western diet.

Patients with pustular acne and low glutathione peroxidase (an antioxidant enzyme) in their red blood cells responded well in one research study to 200 mcg of selenium and 10 mg of alpha tocopherol succinate (a form of vitamin E) twice daily for from 6 to 12 weeks.[1]

More often, patients with acne take one form or another of vitamin A. Retinoic acid, as isotretinoin, is a pharmaceutical derivative of the vitamin that has proven successful for treating severe acne, but not any more successful than the vitamin itself, and both have the same possible danger of causing birth defects when women taking the therapy become unexpectedly pregnant. Other side effects of isotretinoin include problems with adaptation to the dark, staphylococcus aureus infections, aggravation of inflammatory bowel disease, and abnormal growth of bone.

In one study of preformed vitamin A (the actual vitamin, not the drug) used by 136 patients, doses of 300,000 IU for women and from 400,000 to 500,000 IU for men were successful in reducing inflammation, but caused many cases of headaches, nose bleeds, abnormal liver function, and other side effects. Unfortunately, in this study at least, doses below 300,000 IU were ineffective for acne.[2]

Headache may be the first sign of an overdose of vitamin A. One 16-year-old Israeli girl had a headache for a month before doctors realized she was taking a high dose of vitamin A for her acne. After she stopped taking the vitamin, her headache ended.[3] Other symptoms of vitamin A overdose include dry peeling skin, loss of hair, nausea, fatigue, dizziness—in short, overdose is hard to miss. All acute symptoms, other than birth defects, are completely reversible once you stop taking excessive amounts of the vitamin.

Be forewarned. To heal acne and prevent its recurrence, you most likely need to revise your diet (make it very low in fat and sugar, very rich in whole grains, fruits, and vegetables), to adopt a successful means of stress reduction (such as slow breathing, meditation, self-hypnosis, or exercise), and to detoxify your liver using liver-supporting herbs such as milk thistle (silymarin) in addition to nutritional supplements.

Daily Dosage

Vitamin A	50,000 IU for 3 months only
Vitamin C	1 to 3 grams
Vitamin E	400 IU
Brewer's yeast	1 tablespoon twice a day (a good source of minerals)
Selenium	200 mcg
Zinc picolinate	45 mg
Borage oil	3 capsules (a good source of essential fatty acid)
Milk thistle	70 to 210 mg three times a day

.Notes

1. Michaèlsson, G., and Edqvist, L. (1984). Erythrocyte glutathione peroxidase activity in acne vulgaris and the effect of selenium and vitamin E treatment. *Acta Dermato-Venereologica* (Stockholm), 64(1), 9–14. Cited in Werbach, Melvyn R. (1993). *Nutritional Influences on Illness, Second Edition* (p. 9). Tarzana, CA: Third Line Press.

2. Kligman, A. M., et al. (1981). Oral vitamin A in acne vulgaris. *International Journal of Dermatology* 20(4), 278–285. Cited in Werbach, p. 6.

3. Moskowitz, Y., et al. (1993). Pseudotumor cerebri induced by vitamin A combined with minocycline. *Annals of Ophthalmology* 25(8), 306–308.

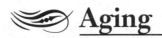 # Aging

What is "old?" An advisory panel of experts was convened in Washington, D.C., to work on problems of the aged. Their first business was to define "aged." They decided it was 10 years older than the oldest among them.

Signs of Aging

It is likely that the experts in Washington had quite a list of physical complaints which they imagined went along with aging: Less hearing, less teeth, less hair, less vision, less memory, less urge for sex; more grey, more joint pain, more waistline, more wrinkles, more mental confusion. Many people believe this prescription for aging is inevitably in their future, if they don't die first of the degenerative diseases characteristic of old age: arthritis, arteriosclerosis, cancer, heart failure, and maturity-onset diabetes. For some, even more foreboding is the specter of senility, and memory loss that isolates affected individuals from those they love.

   While it's probably true that some signs of aging are inevitable, some experts say that much of what we consider normal deterioration isn't due to our age at all. In his book *The Complete Guide to Anti-Aging Nutrients*, Sheldon Saul Hendler cautions that aging has more to do with how we use our years than the number of years we live. Aging, he says, is often the accumulation of affronts we cause to ourselves by smoking, drinking, inactivity, and poor nutrition.[1] I would add to Hendler's list toxins in the environment, including other people's cigarette smoke and also industrial chemicals.

"Our society's misconception is that when you're young and get sick, it's labeled 'illness,' but when you're old and get sick, it's called 'aging.' Sickness and aging, however, are two different states of being," write Abram Hoffer and Morton Walker in *Nutrients to Age Without Senility*.[2] It is important to remember that there are societies in which the diseases we attribute to old age are unknown, even among the elderly.[3] And, what's more, according to the Baltimore Longitudinal Study of Aging (a project of the National Institute on Aging, which began charting the health of more than 1,500 people in 1958), even in our own highly polluted and stressful society some people in their 70s and 80s have healthier cardiovascular systems than some smooth-skinned, greyless 30 year olds.[4]

What this chapter will describe are the ways we unwittingly accelerated the discomforts of old age by increasing the quantity and virulence of free radicals.

What Have Radicals Got to Do with It?

The free radical theory of aging was first suggested in the 1950s by Dr. Denham Harman of the University of Nebraska. Free radicals, those highly excited oxygen atoms with an extra electron, have been described by gerontologist Roy Walford as "great white sharks in the biochemical sea."[5] The predators, as singlet oxygen, hydroxyl radical, or hydrogen peroxide, attack polyunsaturated fats in the membranes surrounding your cells and within the cells. The free radicals also inflict serious damage on proteins and on DNA, which is your unique genetic blueprint found in each cell's nucleus. It is this free-radical-caused damage to genetic material, one theory goes, which is the cause of much of what we call aging.

Smudges on the Blueprint of Life

Your destiny was, in great measure, determined the moment your father's sperm pierced your mother's egg. At that instant, the blue-

Aging

What is it? Aging is not only the accumulation of years, but it is also a gradual mechanical deterioration of body parts and a drop in efficiency of organ function. Some of these changes are inevitable, and some are reversible. The changes of aging result from three major factors: (1) genetic programming, (2) accumulated wear and tear of the immune and endocrine systems in response to dietary, emotional, and environmental factors, and (3) weakened resistance and the breakdown of the body's inherent repair system due to (1) and (2). Just when *old age* begins tends to be a matter of debate, with its beginning defined as happening later and later in life as the age of the person doing the defining advances! Generally, it is considered to begin around 70.

Why is it dangerous? Arthritis, arteriosclerosis, cancer, heart failure, senility, and maturity-onset diabetes are among the debilitating or life-threatening conditions associated with advanced age.

How does it happen? Aging is due to an inevitable rhythm of nature, coupled with the throw of the genetic dice.

print for much of your looks, your talents, your health problems, and the functioning of your various organs was set—not in stone, but in the malleable form of two strips of biological material called phosphate, hung with a sugar and a varying pattern of four bases (a particular kind of chemical compound) facing each other between the strips. Although these two phosphate strips separate entirely when the cell replicates itself, the strips are usually found twisted around each other in a double helix (see Figure 1). This is your DNA. It is found in every cell's nucleus.

Just as the sequence of letters in a sentence makes different words, so the sequence of bases forms a code of genetic inheritance (your *genes*). If the sequence of bases is altered, the message is scrambled. The results can be as minor as a wrinkle or prema-

In addition, excessive free radicals, nutrient deficiencies, food sensitivities, excessive sugar and partially hydrogenated fats, cigarettes, alcohol, lack of exercise, emotional stress, a negative attitude, and a lack of social support all collaborate to wear down the immune system and deteriorate various organs.

What is the effect? Aging is characterized by loss—less hearing, less teeth, less hair, less vision, less memory, less urge for sex—and gain—more grey, more joint pain, more waistline, more wrinkles, more mental confusion.

How can you protect yourself? There is evidence to suggest the benefits of a diet based on vegetables, fruits, whole grains, and seafood, with land animals eaten less often; of a reduced intake of foods with careful attention to the nutritional quality of the foods consumed; of nutritional supplementation with antioxidants (The Four ACES), other nutrients, and selected herbs according to symptoms; of regular aerobic exercise; of involvement in the community and development of a strong support network of friends and family; and of a positive attitude.

turely grey hair, or as major as a birth defect or cancer.

Damage to our genes occurs throughout our life, and, in fact, is a part of the master plan of evolution. These unplanned changes in genes, called *mutations*, allow for the introduction of new features that once in a while are more advantageous to human life than is the status quo. For example, while most people on earth stop producing lactase (the enzyme that digests milk) after about 1 year of age, some northern Europeans' genes mutated to allow continued production of the enzyme. That lead to a population whose intestinal tract felt comfortable consuming dairy products into adulthood. This was an unusual mutation because it was beneficial in terms of survival (a continued supply of protein and calories even when harvests were lean).

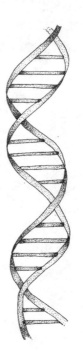

Figure 1 The bars along this double helix of DNA represent the unique sequence of biochemical substances that create your genetic code, dictating much of how you look, act, and feel.

Actually, most genetic mutations are detrimental, and our body quickly acts to correct the mistake. According to the free radical theory of aging, at some point the rate of damage is greater than the rate of repair, and this is what causes aging. Thus, if this theory is true, for an anti-aging drug *par excellence*, scientists need only create a pill that increases the rate of genetic repair. Be assured, they're working on it! Meanwhile, you already have at your fingertips a handy method of decreasing the rate of damage. Antioxidants!

Repairing the Damage

The free radicals that damage DNA are produced not only from exposure to chemicals, radiation, and malnutrition, but also during normal metabolism. Scientists have noticed for about 50 years that free radical levels were higher in aging cells. What they hadn't figured out was whether aging caused free radicals to accumulate in our cells, or vice versa. Then, in early 1994, biologists at Southern Methodist University in Dallas published the results of a genetic experiment with fruit flies that seemed to answer this chicken-or-egg question.

Some lucky fruit flies received extra genes that the researchers knew would clear free radicals out of their cells. The flies lived 30 percent longer and were obviously more active than flies their age with lower levels of antioxidant enzymes. So, staying spritely and alive a good long time seems to boil down to free radical control.[7]

There's quite a difference between looking and feeling great right up to the moment you die, and not dying at all. According to one theory of aging, called the Hayflick hypothesis, we may be able to achieve the former, but it will really be quite a feat to extend what seems to be the human being's maximum life span.

The Hayflick Hypothesis

About 30 years ago, a gerontologist named Leonard Hayflick kept lung tissue cells in bottles of nutrient solution at body temperature. He allowed the cells to divide until they filled the bottles, then threw away half the cells and allowed the rest to keep dividing. When they again filled the bottles, he again threw away half of them and allowed the rest to keep dividing. He called the filling of a bottle by the cell population within it a "doubling," and reported to the scientific community that the cells only doubled 50 times, no matter how he manipulated their conditions.[8]

Further work on what has been termed "the Hayflick limit" has lead many gerontologists to believe in an internal clock, located in a cell's nucleus, that allows the cell, in the best of circumstances, to live a predetermined length of time. The number may not be 50 doublings for all body cells, but the hypothesis is that all healthy body cells have a maximum life span that cannot be exceeded. For example, today the average American man of age 40 can expect to live to around 75. The average American woman of age 40 can expect to live to around 81.[9] A 30 percent increase in longevity (as in the fruit fly experiment) would put our lives still squarely within the 110 to 120 year span that scientists think is the upper limit for human life.[10] (And, by the way, this limit is as high for men as it is for women—men die younger only because of lifestyle factors such as smoking, car accidents, the way they handle stress, and alcoholism; in populations where these factors are nonexistent, such as among the Amish, men live as long as women.)[11]

This upper limit has not changed a bit throughout the history of human life. The difference between the centuries has been a combination of hygiene (especially underground sewers, fewer people in larger living quarters, and clean water) and medical treatment for common infections that formerly decimated populations of the young.

Consequently, humans in the twentieth century have lived past childhood in numbers unheard of in previous centuries. For example, only 33 percent of newborns born in America in 1850 lived past age 60, while at the end of the twentieth century fully 83 percent of us live at least that long. Nevertheless, the longest lived American lives no longer than did the longest lived Roman.[12]

It appears, therefore, that the free radical theory of aging is focused not on creating a biochemical fountain of youth that will allow us to live forever, but rather on allowing us to live as long as we can biologically do so, enjoying a life of vigor and well-being until the day we die (unless those clever scientists find a way to alter the clock before our time is up).

As with most rules, there's an exception: cancer, which totally ignores the Hayflick limit. Cancer cells will keep reproducing as long as they have enough nutrients to keep them alive. Perhaps, in an irony of nature, scientists will find immortality rests within the mystery of the cancer cell, and will harness its power to make Methuselahs of us all.

In the meantime, if we want our cells to last to their full limit of life expectancy, we'd better pay attention to correcting errors that creep into our DNA. The best way to do that is to bathe our cells in all the raw materials they need to function well. That healing nutrient bath begins with what you eat and drink.

Creating a Life of Vigor and Well-Being

In other chapters, you'll read in detail about diets to protect you against heart disease and cancer, the two biggest killers resulting from what you put (or don't put) in your mouth. Here, let's summarize what contemporary research has concluded about the optimum diet for a long and healthy life, a dietary dozen that reduces the amount of free radicals from food and increases the amount of antioxidants and cell nourishment.

1. Cut fat.[13] If you place food on a napkin and it leaves a smear of grease, that's a fatty food you'll want to indulge in only as an occasional treat.

2. Cut partially hydrogenated fats and oils. Boycott cracker and cookie manufacturers who still use these artery-clogging ingredients.[14] Look in the natural foods section of your supermarket for alternatives.

3. When you do eat oil, make it monounsaturated, such as olive oil, or consume a small amount of polyunsaturated vegetable oils and increase your consumption of vitamin E to protect yourself from the easy rancidity of polyunsaturated oil. Avoid frequently eating falafel (balls of chickpeas and spices), churros (long donuts), and other fried fast foods from street vendors who reuse their frying oil for undetermined lengths of time. Reheated oil is a potent source of undesirable free radicals.[15]

4. Cut sugar. Fat and sugar so frequently go together it'll be easier to avoid the one if you are determined to avoid the other. In this way you'll both prevent obesity and leave space on your plate for more vegetables and fruits.

5. Increase the variety and amount of fresh or lightly steamed vegetables. Emphasize the cruciferous vegetables (broccoli, cauliflower, brussels sprouts, cabbage) and those rich in carotene (tomatoes, carrots, squashes, and dark green leafy varieties such as kale, chard, and mustard and collard greens) and vitamin C (potatoes, parsley, green pepper, broccoli, and greens).

6. Increase the variety and amount of fresh fruits, particularly those rich in carotenes (such as cantaloupe and mangoes) and vitamin C (such as strawberries, kiwi, lemons, limes, grapefruit, and oranges).

7. Increase the variety and amount of soy products because they are a source of protein and protect you against cancer.[16] Buy cookbooks that teach you how to use miso soup, tempe, tofu, textured vegetable protein, and other soy foods.

8. Decrease consumption of meat. Some people feel better eating meat, and should continue to eat it, though even they should emphasize lean varieties. It is possible that not everyone is genetically destined to do well as a vegetarian. If you do feel well without meat, cut it out entirely or limit it to special occasions. Just be sure to include protein foods in your diet, such as soy and other beans, and, if you're not a strict vegetarian, eggs (partially hydrogenated oils are more dangerous to your cardiovascular system than are eggs).[17]

9. Limit salt to occasional use. It contributes to high blood pressure and alters the mineral balance in your blood.

10. Eat pickled, smoked, or preserved foods on special occasions only. These foods contribute to cancer of the stomach.[18]

11. Avoid charbroiled or burned food. If you eat it, take an antioxidant supplement to counteract its cancer-causing potential.[19]

12. Avoid eating dyed foods. They can cause allergic reactions in some people.[20] If you must eat such foods, assist your liver in metabolizing these chemicals by increasing your consumption of antioxidants.

Enzyme Power

Antioxidants can be divided into two types: The first is created inside our bodies from the raw materials available. For example, adequate supplies of both vitamin E and selenium are critically important for the activity of glutathione peroxidase, one of the most important enzyme antioxidants.

Other nutritional elements, including the amino acid L-cysteine, can stimulate the activity of glutathione peroxidase. L-cysteine is nontoxic and is an important antioxidant in its own right.

Superoxide dismutase, another powerful enzyme antioxidant, requires sufficient vitamin E, along with copper, manganese, and zinc to sustain its activity. Copper deficiency is rare because the copper in pipes leaches the mineral into your drinking water. But if you rarely eat nuts, fruits, and whole grains, you could easily be consuming too little manganese. Likewise, if your diet is lacking in seeds, seafood, and whole wheat, you could be low in zinc and selenium. By eating these foods, you are assuring your system the ingredients it needs to create the important antioxidant enzymes glutathione peroxidase and superoxide dismutase.

The second type of antioxidant is one that we consume ready-made, either in our food or as a nutritional supplement.

To Supplement or Not to Supplement

Is it enough to follow the dietary dozen shown above? Western medical experts are divided between those who believe you can obtain all the nutrition you need to be healthy from your daily diet and those who believe you will be healthier if you supplement your meals with vitamins, minerals, and other nutrients. One major cornerstone of this controversy is the adequacy or inadequacy of the current RDAs.

RDA stands for Recommended Dietary Allowance. This is the nutrient levels that the United States Food and Drug Administration and the Food and Nutrition Board of the National Academy of Sciences have determined are necessary in the diet of a healthy person to prevent scurvy, pellagra, beri-beri, and other nutritional deficiency diseases.

"The RDA," notes gerontologist Roy L. Walford, "is not slanted toward optimizing modern desires."[21] What Walford means is that what we want today is more than just getting by without nutritional deficiency diseases. We want to prevent cancer and heart disease, to live longer, and look and feel better.

According to an accumulating and impressive body of nutritional research, many of us have a need for some basic nutrients far beyond the RDAs' modest levels.

The RDAs were developed with a hypothetical "average healthy person" in mind. Unfortunately, no one is average and precious few of us are healthy. People who don't fit into the "average" category include people who exercise hard and often, people who are in the hospital, people who have had serious injuries, people who are in convalescent homes, people who are under chronic emotional stress, people who have a family or personal history of birth defects and who want to conceive, people who are on pharmaceutical prescriptions, people who don't eat animal products, and people who are using drugs (including tobacco and alcohol).

Consequently, it behooves you to look at your own individual situation before deciding how much of the essential nutrients you, not the average person, need.

Weakness: A Choice, Not an Inevitability

We usually think of old age and weakness as naturally going together, but when subjects between ages 55 and 74 were given vitamin E at a dose of 727 mg for a month and a half, their ability to run downhill on an incline treadmill for 45 minutes changed from less than to equal to that of a group of subjects between ages 22 and 29.[22] Thus, weakness in the elderly is yet one more result of inadequate nutrition at the cellular level, a result that is, like so many other variables, quickly reversible when the body's cells are appropriately nourished.

Cutting More Than Fat

"Natural antioxidants such as vitamins C and E and beta-carotene, as well as an optimal caloric and protein intake, should be cornerstones of treatment and prevention for the aging patient," writes S. Goldstein of the University of Arkansas.[23] Let's look at this issue of "optimal" caloric and protein intake for slowing aging. What really works using these principles might surprise you!

Although what you put in your stomach is vitally important, what you *don't* consume may be equally so. Fish, rats, mice, and hamsters live longer when they are fed less. Gerontologist Walford of UCLA calls it "undernutrition without malnutrition" and points to experiments in his laboratory with mice that suggest beginning to reduce food intake even in adult humans can help extend life, as long as the human being attempting this technique does so by gradually restricting calories, not suddenly going on a fast.[24]

Back in the Renaissance, a nobleman named Luigi Cornaro spent the first 37 years of his life living out a young man's fantasy, and when his wild lifestyle left him in poor health, he switched to a severely restricted diet and an equally sedate lifestyle for the next 66 years, writing his autobiography, *The Art of Living Long*, and proving he knew of whence he wrote by living to the grand old age of 103 (1464 to 1567).

Why does cutting back on food extend life? "We now think that calorie restriction may extend lifespan by upregulating super-oxide dismutase and catalase," says Walford, explaining that "upregulating" these two antioxidant enzymes performs the same function in us as those new genes did for the lucky experimental fruit flies, described above.[25] It's an efficient, drug-free, surgery-free way to increase the rate our body can eliminate the free radicals that cause us to age.

Walford, in *The 120 Year Diet*,[26] recommends men cut down to about 2,000 nutrient-rich calories per day, and women to 1,800, both adjusting these caloric recommendations to lower levels as they slowly lose weight. Or do as Walford himself does: fast for 2 days a week and eat nourishing foods the other 5 days.

There's More to Long Life Than Antioxidants

Antioxidants are important, but other factors contribute to a healthy body at any age. Primary among these factors is exercise. Ask Luella Tyra, who at age 92 competed in the U.S. Swimming Nationals; or Ada Thomas, who began running for sport at age 65 and ran her first marathon at 68; or Lloyd Lambert, who founded the 70+ Ski Club. And then there's the Over-the-Hill Gang, another elders' ski club whose motto is: "Once you're over the hill, you pick up speed."[27]

Aging causes changes in body composition that include increased fat and decreased bone density. There is a sense of fragility among many old people, for good reason. However, weight-bearing exercise, such as walking, tennis, rope jumping, dancing, or cross country or downhill skiing have increased bone mass in women in their 70s and 80s who started out with fragile bones. And recent research has proven that even at age 96 it is possible to achieve excellent improvement in the size and mass of muscle. How? Lift weights! According to Dr. Joel D. Posner of the Center for Continuing Health at the Medical College of Pennsylvania, weight training is best done with at least a 1-day break in between sessions. Posner cautions older exercisers to stop if they feel chest pain, discomfort, shortness of breath, dizziness, or excessive sweating, particularly if they are also participating in aerobic exercise.[28] Common sense suggests that it is advisable to join an exercise group for these activities, rather than to lift weights or do aerobics at home alone.

Conclusion

Genetic inheritance is certainly important in determining how long we can live, but ensuring that for every year we are alive we are living fully—with zest and good health and passion—has nothing to do with genes and everything to do with the small daily decisions we make about what food and supplements we put in our mouth, what exercise we make time for each week, and how we perceive ourselves in our "old age."

Daily Dosage

If you have specific discomforts, look them up in the later chapter of this book for appropriate advice. For general preventive self-care to counter the effects of aging, the following supplements may be of assistance:

Vitamin A	10,000 IU (or beta-carotene 5,000 IU)
Vitamin C	1–3 grams or to bowel tolerance
Vitamin E	400 IU
Selenium	50 mcg (you may want to take a multimineral that contains this amount of selenium. Take any mineral combination that contains iron at a time of day different from when you take vitamin E, because iron and vitamin E are antagonistic)
Bioflavonoids	1,000 mg
L-cysteine	500 mg twice a day[29]

Notes

1. Hendler, Sheldon Saul. (1983). *The Complete Guide to Anti-Aging Nutrients* (p. 23). New York: Simon & Schuster.
2. Hoffer, Abram, and Walker, Morton. (1980). *Nutrients to Age Without Senility* (p. 28). New Canaan, CT: Keats.
3. Price, Weston. (1945). *Nutrition and Physical Degeneration.* New Canaan, CT: Keats.
4. Hendler, p. 22.
5. Walford, Roy L. (1983). *Maximum Life Span* (p. 87). New York: Norton & Company.
6. Ibid., p. 85.
7. Orr, W. C., and Sohal, R. S. (1994). Extension of life-span by overexpression of superoxide dismutase and catalase in *Drosophila melanogaster. Science* 263(5150), 28–30.
8. Walford, p. 74.
9. Haller, J. (1993). Vitamins for the elderly: Reducing disability and improving quality of life. *Aging Clinical and Experimental Research* 5(Suppl. 1), 65–70.
10. Lin, David J. (1993). *Free Radicals and Disease Prevention* (p. 37). New Canaan, CT: Keats.
11. Walford, p. 18.
12. Walford, p. 4.
13. Kromhout, D. (1992). Dietary fatty acids, serum cholesterol, and 25-year mortality from coronary heart disease: The seven country study. *Circulation* 85, 864.

14. Kromhout, D., and Longnecker, Matthew P. (1993). Do trans acids in margarine and other foods increase the risk of coronary heart disease? *Epidemiology* 4(6), 492–494.

15. Hendler, p. 55.

16. Messina, Mark, and Barnes, Stephen. (1991). The role of soy products in reducing the risk of cancer. *Journal of the National Cancer Institute* 83(8), 541–546.

17. Vorster, Hester H., et al. (1992). Egg intake does not change plasma lipoprotein and coagulation profiles. *American Journal of Clinical Nutrition* 55, 400–410.

18. Weisburger, J. H. (1991). Nutritional approach to cancer prevention with emphasis on vitamins, antioxidants, and carotenoids. *American Journal of Clinical Nutrition* 53, 229S.

19. Hurley, Dan. (1992). Beta-carotene may detoxify carcinogens. *Medical Tribune*, August 20, p. 24.

20. Crook, William G. (1991). *Help for the Hyperactive Child* (pp. 103–105). Jackson, TN: Professional Books.

21. Walford, p. 138.

22. Evans, William J. (1992). Exercise, nutrition and ageing. *Journal of Nutrition* 122, 796–801. Cited in Hamilton, Kirk. (1992). *Clinical Pearls* (p.5). Sacramento, CA: ITServices.

23. Goldstein, S. (1993). The biology of aging: Looking to defuse the genetic time bomb. *Geriatrics* 48(9), 76–82.

24. Walford, pp. 153[en]154.

25. Walford, Roy L. Personal communication, April 14, 1994.

26. Walford, Roy L. (1991). *The 120 Year Diet*. New York: Pocket Books.

27. Dychtwald, Ken, and Flower, Joe. (1990). *Age Wave* (p. 127). New York: Bantam.

28. Posner, Joel D. (1992). Optimal ageing: The role of exercise: A gerontologist who has a center with individualized fitness programs for people over 55 describes the hows and the whys of vigorous exercise—including weight training—for older people. *Patient Care* 26, 35–52.

29. Braverman, Eric R., and Pfeiffer, Carl C. (1987). *The Healing Nutrients Within* (pp. 117–118). New Canaan, CT: Keats.

⮞ Alcoholism

The Egyptians had a brewery back in 3700 B.C., and the Bible refers to wine throughout the holy book, so alcohol has been with us for at least 6,000 years. You'd think a solution to the ails of alcoholism would have been found by now! There may not be an easy solution to stopping alcoholism, but there is a successful way to recover. Although it is one of the best kept secrets in the field of substance abuse, nutritional therapy can eliminate cravings and allow the former abuser to start fresh, feeling good.

The craving for alcohol and many of the symptoms associated with alcoholism are actually signs of specific nutritional deficiencies. The most important nutrients to obtain in the diet and, in many cases, to supplement, include vitamins A, C, and E; the B complex, particularly folic acid and niacin; the amino acid glutamine; and the minerals selenium, zinc, and magnesium.[1]

In Minneapolis, Minnesota, Dr. Joan Mathews Larson has created an alcoholism recovery program with a 75 percent success rate in recovery and maintenance, based on correcting the nutritional deficiencies and biochemical abnormalities that go along with a life on the bottle. Her program detoxifies and nourishes the body from the cells on up. She describes a 7-week self-treatment program in her book *Seven Weeks to Sobriety*.[2]

The Larson program, as practiced at her Health Recovery Center in Minneapolis and described in her book, includes the following elements:

- One week of breaking the addiction, using a detox formula of

18,000 mg of vitamin C in six divided doses per day (reduce by half if diarrhea develops), along with amino acids, a multi-vitamin/mineral combination, additional minerals, a source of essential fatty acids, and pancreatic enzymes to improve absorption of nutrients.

- Four weeks of repairing biochemical damage caused by alcohol, using the detox formula plus flax and a special antioxidant formula of vitamin C, zinc, selenium, glutathione, the antioxidant amino acids methionine and cysteine, vitamin E, coenzyme Q10, and several other lesser antioxidants. Larson also adds milk thistle (silymarin, an antioxidant herb) and a number of other nutrients to promote liver repair and eliminate many of the psychological symptoms of addiction, including poor concentration, angry outbursts, and depression.
- Finding and eliminating food allergies, heavy metal toxicities, thyroid hormone deficiency, *Candida albicans* infection (yeast), and hypoglycemia (low blood sugar).

Daily Dosage

Larson's program changes dosages according to the week of detox and the symptoms. For details, see her book, which can be ordered directly from the author (Bio-Recovery Inc. [800-247-6237] 3255 Hennepin Ave. South, Minneapolis, MN 55426; $14.95 includes shipping and handling).

In addition to Larson's program, there are several other nutritionally oriented alcohol treatment programs in the United States, although none use her protocol. Here is a brief listing of other programs: Health Recovery Center in Minneapolis: 612/827-7800; California Recovery Systems in Mill Valley: 415/383-3611; Milam Recovery Program in Seattle: 206/241-0890; and Comprehensive Medical Care in Amityville, NY: 516/598-2960.

Notes

1. Martin, Paul. (1983). Nutrition and recovery from addiction. *Let's LIVE* January, 67–73.
2. Mathews Larson, Joan. (1993). *Seven Weeks to Sobriety*. New York: Fawcett.

≋ Angina

Angina is pain in the chest that may feel crushing and may radiate outward. It is caused by a lack of oxygen to the heart. People suffering angina have measurable signs of lipid peroxidation in their blood.[1]

In preliminary results from a physician's health study, participants with angina who took 50 mg of beta-carotene every other day for more than 2 years experienced half as many cardiovascular incidents as those taking a placebo.[2] Because of the concern raised by the increased cancer fatalities among those Finnish male smokers taking beta-carotene supplements in a recently published study of nutrient intervention for cancer prevention, beta-carotene is not recommended in high doses at this time. When more research studies are published, we will know beta-carotene's safety record in more detail, and advice may change accordingly. Meanwhile, sticking to high doses of fresh fruits and vegetables is your safest source of beta-carotene.

In another study, patients between the ages of 35 and 54 who had angina were compared to those who did not and were found lacking in vitamins A, C, and E, as well as carotene. The researchers in this 1991 study encouraged the public to include more whole grain cereals, oils rich in vitamin E, vegetables, and fruits in their diet to make use of the protective talents of the antioxidants.[3]

Daily Dosage

Vitamin A   5,000 to 10,000 IU

Vitamin C   Begin with 1 gram and increase dosage to bowel tolerance.

Vitamin E   800 IU for 6 weeks, increasing by 200 IU for the next 6 weeks until results are obtained. This treatment is not recommended for anyone with high blood pressure, and it is recommended that you see your cardiologist for reevaluations at least every 6 weeks while under vitamin E therapy.[4]

Notes

1. Lapenna, Domenico. (1993). Heightened free radical activity in angina pectoris. *The American Journal of Cardiology* 72, 830–831.
2. Gerster, Helga. (1991). Potential role of beta-carotene in the prevention of cardiovascular disease. *International Journal of Vitamin and Nutrition Research* 61, 277–291.
3. Riemersma, R. A., et al. (1991). Risk of angina pectoris and plasma concentrations of vitamins A, C, and E and carotene. *The Lancet* 337(8732), 1–5.
4. Shute, Wilfred E., and Taub, Harald J. (1969). *Vitamin E for Ailing and Healthy Hearts* (p. 46). New York: Pyramid House.

~~~~~ Asthma

Asthma is an allergic reaction of the bronchial tubes that results in a narrowing of the air passages, a swelling of the linings of the tubes, and a filling of the tubes with sticky mucus. The result is difficulty in breathing. Foods, pollens, cats, and other environmental allergens, cold air, exercise, infection, and even emotional distress can trigger asthma. People with asthma are often especially sensitive to food coloring agents and other food additives, such as the sulfites found in wine.

Diet can sometimes contribute to the disease: In one study, 92 percent of 25 patients found significant relief after eliminating all animal foods (meat, fish, poultry, eggs, dairy) for from 4 to 12 months in addition to avoiding chlorinated tap water, chocolate, caffeinated tea, coffee, sugar, and salt.[1]

Antioxidants, including vitamins C and E, the carotenes, and the mineral selenium, are generally considered beneficial for treating asthma and preventing attack, as they protect the lining of the respiratory tract and reduce allergic reactions.

Vitamin C, in particular, can stop the development of an asthma attack (I've used extremely large doses of vitamin C crystals for this purpose). Studies have found that even a dose of 1,000 mg of vitamin C is able to prevent attack in some individuals exposed to asthma triggers.

In one study, subjects taking a daily dose of only 300 mg of vitamin C reported a 30 percent drop in wheezing and bronchial infection.[2] Supplementation of the vitamin is similar to taking an antihistamine drug, because it opens air passages.[3] In fact, vitamin C has commonly been found to be low in people with asthma.

Vitamin C in concert with the amino acid cysteine form an especially powerful combination to open air passages and liquefy mucus, helping to prevent and treat asthma. See "Cysteine" (Part I) for a lengthy description of the use of cysteine and, alternately, a cysteine derivative called NAC, in either aerosol or tablet form, for chronic respiratory conditions.[4]

Bioflavonoids, which are found in nature along with vitamin C (particularly in the white rind of citrus fruit), similarly serve the body as antihistamines and antioxidants. Two herbal sources of these potent antioxidants are green tea and Chinese skullcap (*Scutellaria baicalensis*).[5] Green tea is generally available in any supermarket. You may have to consult an acupuncturist or herbalist for an asthma formula containing Scutellaria. Another herbal source is Ginkgo biloba. In China, in addition to being used to improve brain function, ginkgo has traditionally been used for respiratory conditions such as asthma and bronchitis, probably because flavonoids in the plant's leaves can help reduce inflammation of lung tissues.

Vitamin E, too, has its place in asthma self-care. When 19 adults with asthma took 900 mg of vitamin E each day for several months, they reported a decrease in symptom severity and decreased use of steroid medication.[6]

A study of eight children who suffered frequent respiratory tract infections provided the children 20 mg per kilogram of body weight of vitamin E for 6 weeks. Clinical symptoms subsided, and six of the eight remained healthy during that time.[7]

Daily Dosage

Vitamin A	5,000 to 10,000 IU
Vitamin C	1 to 3 grams or to bowel tolerance
Vitamin E	400 IU
Selenium	250 mcg

Scutellaria   Seek the advice of an herbalist, who will create
                   a formula for you

Ginkgo biloba   240 to 600 mg

Cysteine   200 to 500 mg morning and evening

Decrease these dosages for children in proportion to their weight (an adult weight is generally around 150 pounds, if the child weighs 75 pounds, cut the adult dosages in half).

Notes

1. Lindahl, O., et al. (1985). Vegan diet regimen with reduced medication in the treatment of bronchial asthma. *Journal of Asthma* 22, 45–55.
2. Schwartz, J., and Weiss, S. T. (1990). Dietary factors and their relation to respiratory symptoms. The Second National Health and Nutrition Examination Survey. *American Journal of Epidemiology* 132(1), 67–76.
3. Bucca, C., et al. (1990). Effect of vitamin C on histamine bronchial responsiveness of patients with allergic rhinitis. *Annals of Allergy* 65, 311–314.
4. Braverman, Eric R., with Pfeiffer, Carl C. (1987). *The Healing Nutrients Within: Facts, Findings, and New Research on Amino Acids* (p. 92). New Canaan, CT: Keats.
5. Murray, Michael, and Pizzorno, Joseph. (1991). Asthma and hayfever. *Encyclopedia of Natural Medicine* (pp. 152–153). Rocklin, CA: Prima.
6. Bendich, Adrianne. (1993). Vitamin E and human immune function. *Human Nutrition—A Comprehensive Treatise* Vol. 8, pp. 217–228.
7. Bendich, Adrianne. (1993).

Blindness and Macular Degeneration

Vitamin A deficiency, worldwide, is most often found among preschool children. In acute cases, the conjunctivas of these children dry and ulcerate in a condition called *xerophthalmia*. It is a common cause of blindness among malnourished third world children, blinding about 500,000 youngsters each year.

Xerophthalmia is often accompanied by pneumonia and diarrhea, a deadly combination that kills about 250,000 young children annually.

Community-wide studies in Indonesia and Africa have proven that vitamin A supplementation in these populations can reduce death of young children. For example, a team led by Dr. Alfred Sommer of Johns Hopkins University gave two capsules containing 200,000 IU of vitamin A six months apart to children ages 1 to 5 in Indonesia. There were 229 villages receiving, and 221 not receiving the supplement, with a total of nearly 26,000 children participating. There was a 34 percent reduction in death among the children receiving the vitamin A, compared to controls. According to Sommer, "It is now estimated that improving the vitamin A status of all deficient children worldwide would prevent 1–3 million childhood deaths annually."[1]

In the more developed countries, it is the elderly who share a common cause of blindness called macular degeneration, a deterioration of the macula lutea in the retina that normally allows us to see what is directly in front of us. People suffering macular degeneration cannot see straight ahead, but only vaguely to the edges of their frame of sight.

When researchers at Harvard Medical School compared the diets of people with macular degeneration and those without this condition, they found the higher the amount of beta-carotene in the diet, the lower the risk of this eye condition. This reduced risk was present among former smokers and nonsmokers, but not among those who were currently smoking. In this study, vitamin C also offered reduced risk, but was less effective than vitamin A.[2] In fact, very high doses of vitamin C, coupled with high-energy light focused onto the eye, can actually cause macular degeneration.

The herb Ginkgo biloba has helped people with senile macular degeneration to improve their vision. In one small study of 20 subjects with a randomized, double-blind design, those taking ginkgo for 6 months improved visual acuity in the eye with the least vision by 2.3 diopters while those taking the placebo improved only by 0.6 diopters.[3] Bilberry is another herb that is particularly useful for vision improvement. Read more about this herbal remedy in "Bilberry" (Part I).

Daily Dosage

Vitamin A	5,000 to 25,000 IU
Vitamin C	1 to 3 grams
Vitamin E	400 IU
Ginkgo biloba	180 to 300 mg
Bilberry	60 to 180 mg

Notes

1. Sommer, A. (1993). Vitamin A, infectious disease, and childhood mortality. *Journal of Infectious Diseases* 167(5), 1003–1007.
2. Seddon, J., et al. (1993). Dietary antioxidant status and age related macular degeneration: A multicenter study. *Investigative Ophthalmology and Visual Science* 34, 1134.
3. Lebuisson, D. A., et al. (1986). Treatment of senile macular degeneration with Ginkgo biloba extract: A preliminary double-blind study versus placebo. *Presse Medicine* 15, 1556–1558. Cited in Murray, Frank. (1993). *Ginkgo Biloba* (p. 35). New Canaan, CT: Keats.

~~~> Burns

Each year at least 2 million people in the United States suffer severe burns requiring medical attention. A burn can be caused by many different sources of heat, including hot water, hot metal (such as iron), electricity, or open flames. Electrical burns don't always show on the skin surface and require special attention by a physician. Burns on the skin's surface can be first degree (only the uppper layers are damaged, as in a sunburn), second degree (damage deep enough to cause blisters, but the deepest layers of skin are left undamaged), or third degree (every layer is affected, and medical treatment is required to prevent serious scarring and contraction).

A burn patient needs extra vitamin C because the vitamin is particularly adept at creating new collagen, the connective tissue that is damaged when the skin is burned.[1] Some researchers suggest 500 mg of vitamin C per day, with half that dosage given to children.[2]

Vitamin A is also suggested for its role in maintaining health of the skin. Extrapolating from a study of burned guinea pigs, some researchers suggest from 10,000 to 100,000 IU of vitamin A daily following burn injury, or three liters per day of 20,000 IU vitamin A per liter intravenously, which they believe would be therapeutic without being toxic.[3]

In *Vitamin E for Ailing and Healthy Hearts*, Dr. Wilfrid E. Shute describes the benefits of vitamin E taken internally. A child age 6 suffered second degree burns to his fingers from a hot laundry iron, and since at the time there was no topical vitamin E preparation available, the boy was given 300 IU of alpha tocopherol by mouth daily. He regained complete function of the hand, healing was rapid, there was no infection or deepening of the damaged tissue, and he needed no skin grafting.

Externally, vitamin E is the premier treatment for burns, whether they are simple or serious. Another 6-year-old patient of Shute's suffered multiple burns from boiling water, and skin grafting was unsuccessful. He was in the hospital with grossly infected areas over his neck, back, chest, and left thigh. There was no evidence of healing even weeks after the accident. Vitamin E ointment was applied directly to the wound (alternated with antibiotic ointment for the first 10 days), and the boy was given 300 IU of alpha tocopherol by mouth daily. The infection cleared in 4 days, and the wound completely healed in 13 weeks without needing skin grafting and without the scar tissue contracting or keloiding.

Shute describes several adults with similar good results from topical treatment of severe burns with vitamin E ointment, including one woman with second and third degree burns on her arms, chest, and thigh from boiling water who was told by a large metropolitan hospital that she would need extensive grafting. Instead, she signed out and moved in with her daughter. Visiting nurses dressed her wounds with alpha tocopherol ointment on gauze. Three months and 27 pounds of ointment later, at the time the book was written, all areas except the most severe burn on one arm had healed without contraction or scar tissue. The remaining unhealed area on her arm was still being dressed with ointment daily.

Daily Dosage

Vitamin A	10,000 to 100,000 IU, orally or 3 liters per day of 20,000 IU vitamin A per liter administered intravenously
Vitamin C	500 mg or bowel tolerance
Vitamin E	300 to 400 IU orally and continual dressing of the wound with vitamin E as an ointment or oil until healed

Notes

1. Dylewski, D. F., and Froman, D. M. (1992). Vitamin C supplementation in the patient with burns and renal failure. *Journal of Burn Care and Rehabilitation* 13(3), 378–380. See also Pasulka, Patrick S., and Wachtel, Thomas L. (1987). Nutrition considerations for the burned patient. *Surgical Clinics of North America/Burns* 67(1), 109–131. Cited in Hamilton, Kirk. (1990). *Clinical Pearls* (p. 80). Sacramento, CA: ITServices.

2. Waymack, J. Paul, and Herndon, David N. (1992). Nutritional support of the burned patient. *World Journal of Surgery* 16, 80–86. Cited in Hamilton, Kirk. (1992). *Clinical Pearls* (p. 99). Sacramento, CA: ITServices.

3. Kuroiwa, K., et al. (1990). Effect of vitamin A and enteral formulae for burned guinea-pigs. *Burns* 16(4), 265–272. Cited in Hamilton (1990), p. 81.

4. Shute, Wilfrid E., and Taub, Harald J. (1969). *Vitamin E for Ailing and Healthy Hearts* (pp. 164–169). New York: Pyramid House.

～⁓ Cancer

Perhaps you live in a highly polluted city, are addicted to cigarettes, live with someone who smokes, or work with toxic chemicals. Before you throw your hands up in despair, take a deep breath (yes, even of the air where you live). I can't guarantee you'll be free of cancer, but be assured there's a lot you can do to protect yourself from it.

You can begin, of course, by stopping smoking. Short of that, you can begin to eat with vitamins and minerals in mind: There is a significant difference in the risk of cancer between smokers who do and who do not pay attention to daily nutrition.[1]

A Closer Look at Cancer

It is important to remember that all of us throughout our lives develop abnormal cells that could become or already have become cancerous. These abnormal cells are destroyed by our immune system before they cause us damage. Everyone who has been treated for cancer and whose disease has "gone into remission" has managed to restimulate his or her own inner defense team to do its protection work. Destroying cancer cells is an everyday, unspectacular function of our immune system, *when it has the tools to do the job.*

Cancer

What is cancer? Cancer can be described as cells reproducing at an abnormally high rate.

Why is it dangerous? Cell overgrowth can interfere with normal body functions to the point of irreparable damage, and even death.

What else is it called? Cancer is also called neoplasia, meaning "new form." A malignant metastatic *neoplasia* is an overgrowth of cells that seeds itself at sites distant from its original site.

How does it happen? The immune system's normal ability to seek out and destroy abnormal cells is thwarted, due to a combination of factors relating to emotions, heredity, environmental pollution, smoking, and nutritional deficiencies.

What is the effect? Depending on the site and the extent of cancer, affected organs gradually lose their function and whole systems shut down.

We make staying free of cancer more difficult when we get in the way of our own defense team. For example, we may drink alcohol to excess, smoke cigarettes, or continually expose ourselves to industrial chemicals and radiation. To stay healthy we must provide our defense team the tools it needs to do its work. These tools include a positive, assertive attitude[2]; a healthy lifestyle; and nutrients of various kinds that enhance our immune system. There are also inside defenders called superoxide dismutase, catalase, and glutathione peroxidase that we produce from good eating habits. And we must not forget the antioxidant nutrients: vitamins A, C, and E, and the mineral selenium, which we obtain directly from the food we eat.

Both the inside defenders and the defenders found in food are

What can you do to protect yourself?

- Eat a minimum of five fruits and vegetables each day; when possible, choose produce grown without pesticides and herbicides.
- *Don't smoke cigarettes* and avoid exposure to secondhand smoke.
- Drink clean water free of industrial chemicals.
- Prevent hidden nutritional deficiencies by taking supplemental antioxidants.
- Drink commercial black or green tea, which contain antioxidant substances called polyphenols.
- Maintain an optimistic outlook and insist on participating in all decisions related to your health.

How can you obtain additional protection? Take supplemental minerals such as calcium, magnesium, and zinc; and boost your intake of vitamin D and the vitamin B complex, particularly folic acid.

helped by essential minerals that are also found in food, such as calcium, magnesium, zinc, vitamin D, and folic acid (one of the B complex vitamins).

Just the Facts

Cancer rates are rising in the industrialized world, probably because of cigarette use. A recent Swedish study found that "baby boomers" face a higher risk of cancer than their grandparents did. In one study, cancer was found to be almost three times as prevalent among men born in the 1950s compared to men born in the 1880s! Something's changed in the span of two generations and the change isn't good.

In the United States, as well, cigarettes are a major cause of cancer, but cigarette use among men has been dropping, while there has been a 55 percent increase in cancer among men (and a 30 percent rise in cancer among women) since 1958. Overall, about one in every three Americans will be diagnosed with cancer in his or her lifetime.[3]

Whatever the cause, lung, pancreas, kidney, brain, and breast cancers have all been increasing in frequency during the past 40 years.[4]

Critics of cancer research and treatment claim the current emphasis is too great on pharmaceuticals that are both expensive and dangerous, and too little on prevention. For example, cancer rates would plummet, these researchers say, if the public was vigorously encouraged to eat more antioxidant-rich fruits and vegetables and less fat, salt, and sugar; to eliminate tobacco use; and to severely restrict exposure to cancer-causing chemicals and radioactive substances.[5] (Since changing eating habits can happen overnight, unlike a change in the health of our environment, it is comforting to know that carotenes in fruits and vegetables can help protect you against even cancer-causing industrial waste.)[6]

What Is Cancer?

Cancer basically means cells that refuse to behave. Directions as to what cells look like, how they will develop, and how many times they will reproduce are coded into the structure of a cell's DNA (the basic genetic material in a cell's nucleus). Sometimes, toxic substances like viruses, chemicals, radiation, and free radicals attack and alter DNA. This is called the *initiation* stage of cancer. In it faulty directions are created on how the cell must grow. Next comes the *promotion* stage of cancer. The cell begins following these new, incorrect, directions, and, like a photocopier gone wild, reproduces uncontrollably. This wild reproduction is fostered by "cancer promoters" such as excess estrogens or bile acids.

Cancer cells may migrate (doctors say *metastasize*) through the blood and lymph to distant sites and continue their wildly untamed reproduction there, as well. This is called a malignancy, and at this stage the cancer is life threatening unless something comes along to stop the uncontrolled reproduction, eliminate cancerous cells, and fine-tune the DNA of abnormal cells to correct those misdirections.

Time to Intervene

Regardless of the specific initiator or promoter, cancer develops over time and through a number of different stages. It may take as many as five or more discrete changes in a cell's DNA for cancer cells to become malignant, and as long as *ten* or *twenty* years from initiation to promotion, which is one reason cancer most often occurs in older people.[7]

To be more specific, cancer doesn't appear the first time you step out of a plane and inhale the smoggy air in Los Angeles, or sit in a smoky cocktail lounge, or work within an electromagnetic field, or are covered by aerial-sprayed pesticide. However, you must do something extra to protect yourself if you're a resident of Los Angeles or other smoggy towns, a bartender, a telephone lineman,[8] or a farmworker,[9] because the most dangerous situation is when you are continually exposed to *carcinogens* (substances that cause the development of cancer).

"It has been estimated that about 75–80 percent of all human cancers are environmentally induced, about 35 percent with smoking and 35 to 40 percent of them by diet," says Dr. John H. Weisburger of the American Health Foundation in New York.[10] Other researchers suggest diet is involved in as many as *60 percent* of cancers.[11] Imagine! More than a half of cancers are directly related to what we choose to put in our mouths! Even smokers, who inhale over 4,000 chemicals including many carcinogens and cancer promoters in every puff, show a different risk for cancer depending simply on how many fruits and vegetables they include in their daily diet.[12]

Diet as Self-Protection

When it comes to cancer prevention, look inside your own refrigerator and if you're storing fruits and vegetables there, rejoice. Of more than 100 human studies, 93 percent show those who regularly eat fruits and vegetables, particularly yellow and green vegetables and cruciferous vegetables in the *Brassica* family (brussels sprouts, cauliflower, cabbage, and broccoli), have a lower likelihood of developing cancer than similar people who don't eat vegetables.

In the summer of 1988, in fact, the state of California launched a "5 a Day for Better Health" campaign to encourage adults to eat at least five fresh fruits and vegetables each day.[13] The National Cancer Institute followed California's example, opening its own "5 a Day" campaign in the summer of 1992. The need was obvious. Surveys show that about three out of four children in America eat fewer than five servings of produce during any 2-day period.[14] And, on any given day, only 9 percent of American adults consume five or more fruits and vegetables.[15]

A deficiency of the antioxidants found in yellow and green vegetables and fruits isn't the only dietary causes of cancer. A high-fat, high-calorie, low-fiber diet contributes to your risk for cancer of the breast, bladder, kidneys, colon and rectum, prostate, ovary, endometrium (womb), and pancreas. Yet, even among meat eaters, those who eat the most vegetables have a lower risk of cancer than those who don't eat vegetables.

Take Tea

In addition to consuming *lots* more vegetables and fruits, you can start drinking green or black tea as part of your prevention program. Green and black tea are from the plant *Camellia sinensis*. They contain polyphenols, antioxidant biochemicals that protect the body from developing cancer by inhibiting proliferation of cells and by blocking the formation of *N*-nitroso compounds. They particularly protect us from the carcinogens called heterocyclic amines produced from cooking meat (so if you insist on charcoal broiling your steak, you may want to have a nice cup of tea with it!).[16]

In Japan, the people of Shizuoka Prefecture, where green tea is a staple product, die significantly less from cancer of all sites than other citizens of Japan. For stomach cancer, particularly, mortality was much lower among those Japanese drinking green tea compared to Japanese drinking other beverages.

Not all studies show a clear 100 percent connection between tea consumption and reduction of cancer at all sites; however, laboratory studies do clearly indicate that tea can inhibit the development of tumors.

Use the following diet recommendation to prevent cancer of the breast, bladder, cervix, colon, lung, mouth and oral cavity, pancreas, prostate, rectum, stomach, and uterus[17]:

Decrease	Increase
Pickled foods	Fiber
Smoked foods	Fruit
Alcohol	Vegetables
Nitrites, nitrates	Soy products
Meat	Legumes
Fat	Garlic, berries, green or black tea, whole grains, fish

What's So Special about Vegetables?

What's in vegetables that keeps cancer from developing? The list includes carotenes, vitamins C and E, selenium, flavonoids, phenols, indoles, folic acid, glutathione, fiber, plant sterols, and at least six other biochemicals. For this reason, the search for "the" substance to prevent cancer is doomed to fail. Nature does not work that way! These natural substances in vegetables (and fruits, too) overlap in their effects and complement each other.

Kristi Steinmetz and John D. Potter, in an article on the subject of foods and cancer prevention, suggest cancer may be a disease created by the body in response to deficient consumption of foods that are needed to maintain health.[18] Together, these nutritional substances form the "anticarcinogenic cocktail" which creates detoxifying enzymes, stops the creation of cancerous cells, dilutes and binds cancer-causing substances in the digestive tract, supports antioxidant activities, and forms the basis for the creation of our most successful cancer-prevention defense team.

Vitamin A, Beta-Carotene, and Cancer

Vitamin A is able to inhibit the growth of tumor cells and to help one cell talk to a nearby cell and keep them developing along the same line. Along with vitamin E, it can also control the expression of certain genes that might direct cells to become actively cancerous.

For 25 years, research has accumulated evidence linking vitamin A, beta-carotene, and a second carotene, called lycopene, with lowered risk of cancer. The basis for this relationship seems logical: cancer cells are stuck in an unfinished stage of development and keep reproducing themselves in this immature stage. Along comes vitamin A and the carotenes and together they nudge these recalcitrant cells into maturing normally.

Inside certain fruits and vegetables is a biological compound called beta-carotene. Beta-carotene is known for its ability to transform itself into vitamin A inside our body. Amazingly, only as much beta-carotene transforms into vitamin A as we need at that time. Some percent of untransformed beta-carotene remain intact in the bloodstream and work as an anti-tumor force, stopping the initiation and the promotion of cancer in selected tissues.

One of the most surprising food and cancer studies came out of Israel back in 1981, showing a very significant benefit of tomatoes against gastrointestinal cancer.[19] Tomatoes have almost no beta-carotene, but are high in the carotene called lycopene. Lycopene does not convert into vitamin A in the body. It apparently has its own unique ability to fight cancer on a grand scale.

Just before this book was completed, one lone but well-designed study of smokers in Finland concluded that those taking supplemental beta-carotene actually developed cancer at a higher rate than those not taking the supplement.[20] This is the opposite result of numerous epidemiological reports comparing cancer rates with diet that have been published recently. Consequently, the scientific community (and the rest of us) are waiting for the results of several other beta-carotene studies currently underway to explain this anomaly. Until the issue is settled, it is safest to obtain beta-carotene by increasing the number of fruits and vegetables you eat daily, instead of obtaining it from supplements. After all, one medium carrot will supply you with about 7,900 IU of beta-carotene, and one cup of cooked spinach offers 15,000 IU! Supplement takers may want to stick with 3 mg (5,000 IU), as found in various multivitamins.

Vitamin C and Bioflavonoids

In 1990, the National Cancer Institute (NCI) invited researchers to Bethesda, Maryland, to share their work with vitamin C in the international fight against cancer. Dr. Gladys Block, who is currently professor of public health, nutrition, and epidemiology at the University of California, Berkeley, reviewed all studies of vitamin C against cancer of the oral cavity, esophagus, larynx, lung, breast, stomach, pancreas, bladder, cervix, endometrium (uterus), colon, and rectum, and also childhood brain tumors. She found 34 out of 47 studies suggested the vitamin protected those sites at a dose of about 380 mg per day.[21] At the same symposium, Dr. Balz Frei of Harvard University reported that no cancer-causing chemical reactions could be detected in human blood plasma as long as vitamin C was present, but when vitamin C was lacking, lipid peroxidation (which is believed to be a cause of cancer) resumed.[22]

Researchers in one study looked at the relationship between vitamin C consumption and death from cancer and other causes in a group of over 11,000 Americans ages 25 to 74. They examined the group between 1971 and 1974. For the men studied, those who took the most vitamin C were most likely to still be alive 10 years later. The connection between vitamin C and longevity was there but was weaker for women.[23]

Bioflavonoids have also been found useful, along with other nutritional substances in fruits and vegetables, to prevent cancer at many sites.[24]

Selenium and Cancer

And then there's selenium. Research suggests that consuming from 50 to 200 mcg of selenium daily can prevent most cancers.[25] Some Americans obtain less than these protective doses in their daily diet, even though rich sources such as seafood, whole wheat, oatmeal, brown rice, and organ meats (such as liver and kidney) are widely available.

Antioxidants Plus Drugs

Combination chemoprevention is the hottest new health-care idea among Western researchers. It means combining several therapies to improve outcome and to reduce unwanted side effects. It is a concept used for the past 4,000 years in Chinese herbal formulas, which usually involve combining as many as a dozen different plant and animal substances to counteract each other's deficiencies and toxicities.

In the West, oncologists have recently discovered the benefits of combining tamoxifen, an anti-cancer agent, and retinoids, a form of vitamin A. One particular retinoid, called fenretinide [4-(N-hydroxyphenyl)retinamide] concentrates in the breast and, like tamoxifen, increases the activity of a part of the immune system which reins in runaway cell reproduction.[26]

Retinoids, however, have their own toxicities. In a perfect example of combination chemoprevention, vitamin E has been used to cut the side effects of retinoid therapy, which has been used to enhance the outcome of conventional therapy for lymphoid cancer! Another example is using cysteine, either as an amino acid or as a patented version called N-acetylcysteine (NAC), along with cyclophosphamide.[27] When patients took four times as much NAC as cyclophosphamide a half hour before chemotherapy, they did not suffer the inflammation and bleeding of the bladder that often accompanies cyclophosphamide use. European studies using a drug comparable to cyclophosphamide also found that patients were protected from severe side effects by employing similar supplementation.[28]

NAC as a skin ointment protected patients from hair loss, damage to the mucous membranes of the eyes, and skin damage from radiation therapy.[29]

Other examples of combination chemoprevention are doxorubicin (Adriamycin®) and cysteine, and Adriamycin and coenzyme Q10.

Cosmetically speaking, supplementing daily with 1,600 IU of

vitamin E in the form of dl-alpha tocopherol acetate the week before receiving Adriamycin prevented hair loss in 69 percent of patients in one study.[30] Those who did lose their hair were believed to have been given the supplement too late before chemotherapy began. Researchers advise the best time to take the vitamin is at least 5–7 days prior to beginning chemotherapy.

You can expect the discovery of many more examples of such collaboration between pharmacological agents and antioxidants in the near future.

Beware the Magic Bullet Mentality

The antioxidants discussed here are very important, but at this time in medical history, we don't know all the nutrients that are found in nature, let alone all the nutrients that are important cancer preventive agents.

For example, in the February/March 1994 issue of the *Townsend Letter for Doctors*, columnist Dr. Alan R. Gaby describes a new study by Japanese researchers on cancer-fighting flavonoids found in plant foods. The Japanese found that one flavonoid, *genistein*, stopped the growth of human stomach cancer cells in their test tubes.[31] Genistein is found in soy products.

"As the present study indicates," warns Gaby, "plant foods also contain lesser known compounds that possess potent biological activity. Although taking supplements is probably helpful, there is no substitute for the real food."

Special Considerations of Children

As we invent more and better recipes to interest our children in the "V" word (vegetable), a nagging worry remains: How will our children be affected by the increased exposure to herbicides and pesticides in those carotene-rich fruits and vegetables?

In June 1993, the National Academy of Sciences (NAS) released a report titled *Pesticides in the Diets of Infants and Children* that pointed out that children react to toxic chemicals, including pesticides, in different ways than do adults, and in some cases are more sensitive to such toxins than are adults.

The NAS report could find no documented case where legal use of pesticides specifically caused illness. In fact, according to Dr. Bruce N. Ames, "There are about 10,000 different natural pesticides in our diet, and they usually are present at enormously higher levels than synthetic pesticides."[32] Ames, a professor of biochemistry and molecular biology at the University of California, Berkeley, and a world-renown toxicologist, believes the three major causes of cancer are smoking; too much fat and calories in our diet and too little fruit, vegetables, fiber, and calcium; and chronic inflammations such as hepatitis and parasites. He, and many other researchers, think the public's fear of pesticides is unrealistic.

So, what's a conscientious parent to do? One answer is to live a lifestyle that incorporates cancer protection into it on a daily basis. Five fruits and vegetables a day are a minimum. The more the better. Buy organic food when it is available. Support farmer's markets in your town, and talk to the farmers themselves to let them know you prefer food grown without pesticides and herbicides. Grow your own vegetables. Clean your food carefully of external chemical residues. Remember, the fruits and vegetables contain cancer-fighting beta-carotene and vitamin C, along with many other important nutrients, so nature has provided built-in protection for you. And, make sure that whatever you eat is consumed in an atmosphere of love and respect for the effort of all those who grew it, picked it, transported it, sold it, prepared it, and are sharing it at that meal.

Where Do We Go from Here?

In choosing a path to take, we might listen to the medical researchers themselves. "The question," said Dr. Jeffrey B. Blumberg, Chief of the Antioxidants Research Lab at Tufts University, "must be 'What is the effect of the person's antioxidant status?', rather than the status of each one." It is, in other words, the combination of antioxidants that offers us the most health benefits. Gerald Shklar of the Harvard School of Dental Medicine agrees, noting antioxidants work synergistically, their mix more powerful

than any one alone. Said Shklar at a November 1993 FDA conference on Antioxidant Nutrients and Cancer and Cardiovascular
Disease, "I really have no doubt that most human cancers will be
prevented or regress if we get antioxidants to the tumors." Note
the plural.

Research-oriented government agencies like the National
Cancer Institute aren't yet ready to give the public a blanket sug-
gestion to take nutritional supplements, though they are encour-
aging us all to eat more fruits and vegetables. Individual
researchers are more enthusiastic about nutritional supplements.
As Blumberg said, "the probability of benefit is good, and the
potential for side effects and toxicity is low." At bottom, however,
is a unanimous agreement that a diet well balanced in antioxidants
is the most important first step to prevent cancer. And if you
choose to supplement your meals, take the full spectrum of The
Four ACES. If we want to improve on nature, we have to start by
mimicking nature, and nature works her nutrients one with
another in a synergistic symphony of defense and nourishment.

Daily Dosage

For vitamin A, studies of patients undergoing chemotherapy and
radiation have used 15,000–40,000 IU per day to prevent side
effects. (This dose is for a limited time only.) In general, a dose of
5,000–10,000 IU per day is safe, though with vitamin A, since it is
stored in the liver and fat cells, each person's· level of toxicity is
unique.

For beta-carotene, 3 mg per day (5,000 IU) is considered a
reasonable dose, though this may change in the coming years as
more research is completed.

For vitamin C, begin with 250 mg per day. If you are exposed
to toxins from cigarettes, smog, chemicals, or infection, up the
dose according to bowel tolerance. (Take only as much as won't
cause your bowels to loosen. See "Vitamin C and Bioflavonoids"
for more specific directions on bowel tolerance doses.)

For vitamin E, studies generally find positive results at
100–400 IU per day.

Individual Cancer Sites
and Antioxidant Therapy

Following are individual cancer sites and selected medical research on antioxidant protection and treatment for each site.

Bladder

Approximately 49,000 persons in the United States develop bladder cancer each year. Moderate to heavy smokers show a two- to five-fold risk of bladder cancer, compared to those who never smoked. Another cause of bladder cancer is exposure to aromatic amines in the workplace. In fact, certain professions appear particularly at risk for bladder cancer, such as dye workers, rubber workers, leather workers, painters, truck drivers, and aluminum workers.[33]

Fruits, vegetables, and foods high in preformed vitamin A (such as liver and fish) seem to offer some protection against bladder cancer.

In terms of treatment, one recent study gave 35 patients with bladder cancer 40,000 IU of vitamin A, 100 mg of B-6, 2,000 mg of vitamin C, and 400 IU of vitamin E along with conventional therapy. Only 40 percent of these patients developed new tumors, compared with 80 percent of 30 patients given conventional therapy alone. In addition, although about 75 percent of both groups survived, of those who did die, survival time was 33 months in the supplemented group, compared to 18 months in the unsupplemented group.[34] Dr. Michael Jewett, chairman of urology at the University of Toronto, told an interviewer he would tell any bladder cancer patient who wanted to try vitamins "there do not seem to be any harmful effects and there may be some benefit."

Breast

Breast cancer is the most frequently diagnosed malignancy among women, and has increased at least 57 percent since 1950.[35]

New research suggests that environmental assaults, from radiation, PCBs (*polychlorinated biphenyls*, a family of industrial chemicals), and pesticides are possibly important causes of breast cancer.[36]

"Perhaps," suggests J. H. Hankin of the University of Hawaii's Cancer Research Center, "no area is more controversial than the link between . . . dietary fat and the development of breast cancer."[37] In 1990, one investigator named Geoffrey R. Howe reviewed 12 studies of diet and breast cancer and found a significant connection between increased risk for the disease and increased consumption of saturated fat, particularly among postmenopausal women. The problem is, there have been other studies with conflicting results. Nevertheless, Howe suggests that if indeed a high-fat diet contributes to breast cancer, then by lowering the fat in our diet we in North America could prevent 24 percent of breast cancers in postmenopausal women, and 16 percent in premenopausal women.[38] Lest you throw out all the fat and oil in your household, Dr. John H. Weisburger of the American Health Foundation points out that olive oil does not increase breast cancer risk and fish oils help protect you from cancer.[39]

No Recurrence with Vitamin A. What about vitamins? In 1980, Harvard researchers questioned over 89,000 women as to their diet and supplement use. They reassessed the women's consumption of nutrients in 1984. Then, 8 years later, they looked at the women who had subsequently developed breast cancer and found that those with the highest vitamin A consumption had the lowest risk of developing the disease. In contrast, vitamins C and E did not seem to protect the women from breast cancer.[40]

When University of Illinois at Chicago researchers measured the amount of vitamin A in the blood of women who underwent both a mastectomy and chemotherapy, they found those with the higher concentrations of retinol-binding protein, the main carrier of vitamin A in the blood, were the most likely to be free of cancer 2 years later. Those with low levels of this marker of vitamin A status were more likely to have had fibrocystic breast disease before their diagnosis of cancer and more likely to have metastatic growths of cancer beyond the original site in the breast.[41]

Vitamin C for Breast Health. In conclusion, to help protect yourself from breast cancer, work politically for a clean environment and make sure your daily diet is low in fat and rich in fruits and vegetables. Antioxidant supplementation may also help.

Cervix

The cervix is the opening to the womb or uterus. Women with genital warts or genital herpes infections and those who smoke cigarettes are at greater risk for cervical cancer than is the general population. There is a greater incidence of cervical cancer in the developing world that in the industrialized world. In the West, lower socioeconomic groups have more cervical cancer than wealthier populations. Inadequate hygiene may be one cause, although nutrition may also play a role.

Women with abnormalities of the cervix have lower levels of vitamins A and C than do women with normal cervixes. Conversely, high intake of yellow and green vegetables, which are rich in these two vitamins, may offer some protection. There are intervention trials currently underway that will give us clearer information on this diet–cancer connection.

Even before cancer begins, women may have abnormal changes in their cervix, called *dysplasia*. One research team had women with moderate dysplasia use the form of vitamin A called isotretinoin (12-*cis*-retinoic acid) in their cervical caps (a barrier form of contraception that sits snugly around the cervix). This treatment improved the dysplasia in 80 percent of the women in this study.[42]

Colon and Rectum

Colon cancer is the second most common cause of death from cancer in the United States. It is a disease peculiar to the Western world. Thus, some researchers claim that 90 percent of colon cancer deaths might be caused by our diet, particularly by our emphasis on meat and fat and our slighting of whole grains and vegetables.[43] For example, when Japanese city dwellers adopted a more Western, high-fat diet, their incidence of colon cancer increased.[44]

Bile acids, produced by the liver and by intestinal bacteria, seem to be an important element in the promotion of colorectal cancer. The amount of fat in our diet controls the amount of bile acids that are formed. Vegetables and cereals that add bulk to the diet inhibit the formation of these bile acids and help protect us from cancer of the bowel. Not only does increased vegetable and cereal fiber dilute potentially toxic contents of the bowel, it also shortens the time the waste moves through our intestine, shortening our exposure to the toxic substances in the stool.

Not all studies show a clear connection between fat intake and increased risk of bowel cancer. However, the relationship between fiber and bowel cancer is consistent. In fact, one group of Canadian researchers estimate that 50,000 fewer cases of colorectal cancer would occur in the United States alone if we significantly increased our consumption of fiber.[45] Another risk factor may be alcohol consumption.[46]

Recent evidence points to antioxidants, particularly vitamin E, as well as other nutritional elements (such as calcium and vitamin D) as able to help protect against bowel cancer development. For example, researchers interviewed over 35,000 Iowa women in 1984, then compared the diets of the 212 women who developed colon cancer by 1990 with the diets of women who hadn't developed cancer. A high intake of vitamin E seemed to be protective, especially in women under age 65.[47]

You can obtain both fiber and vitamin E in one package, if you increase your consumption of 100 percent whole wheat products. In addition, increase your consumption of vegetables, because this will add not only vegetable fiber but also a hefty complement of beta-carotene as well. And that's a good idea since the liver transforms beta-carotene to vitamin A, and vitamin A is essential both for the health of the cells lining the colon and to help cells that are beginning to wildly reproduce themselves to start acting normal.[48]

Leukemia

One of the most stunning successes of antioxidants in cancer treatment was announced to the world in 1988 by Chinese scientists who claimed remissions of acute promyelocytic leukemia followed the use of a form of vitamin A (all-trans retinoic acid).[49] Researchers have since used other derivatives of vitamin A for other forms of leukemia.[50] Scientists have known for more than 50 years that derivatives of vitamin A, called retinoids, can control the reproduction and the differentiation of cells. It took time, however, for someone to apply that knowledge to cases of leukemia. What seems to work best is a combination of chemotherapy and retinoid therapy, since retinoid therapy alone has proven to have only temporary success.

Lung

Lung cancer is clearly associated with smoking cigarettes, yet smokers who consume high levels of vitamin A and beta-carotene have a lower incidence of lung cancer than those who don't eat their fruits and vegetables.[51] In fact, several studies have shown that people with lung cancer report eating fewer foods rich in vitamin A and beta-carotene than do people without lung cancer.[52]

Apart from cigarettes, up to 40 percent of lung cancer may be attributable to exposure to carcinogenic substances at work.[53] In addition, the nitrogen dioxide in smog is dangerous to lungs, and researchers find a noticeable drop in antioxidant levels in the human lung when exposed to smoggy days or cigarette smoke.[54]

When doctors used antioxidants along with radiation and chemotherapy for small-cell lung cancer, patients lived longer (44 percent were still alive with a mean survival time of 32 months by the end of the study), and tolerated radiation and chemotherapy better than the group not given antioxidants. In this study, patients were given daily doses ranging, according to individual need, from 15,000 to 40,000 IU of vitamin A; 10,000 to 20,000 IU of beta-carotene; 300 to 800 IU of vitamin E; 2,000 to 5,000 mg of vitamin C; and 856 to 3,424 mcg of selenium in the form of sodium selenate. They were also given from 97 to 194 mg of manganese.[55]

We will know a lot more about the relationship between beta-carotene and lung cancer when researchers publish the results of an important study currently underway. The study is, wouldn't you know it, titled CARET (for Carotene and Retinol Efficacy Trial) and is looking at two populations at high risk for lung cancer: asbestos-exposed workers and heavy smokers. Nearly 18,000 participants in Seattle, Portland, San Francisco, Irvine, Baltimore, and New Haven are taking a daily combination of 30 mg of beta-carotene and 25,000 IU of vitamin A as retinyl palmitate. Initial results are expected in 1998.

Oral Cavity and Esophagus

In 1989, there were more than 30,000 new oral cavity cancer cases in the Unites States. These include the mouth, larynx, and pharynx. I am also adding the esophagus to this category. Epidemiological research has found blood levels of vitamin A, beta-carotene, and vitamin B-2 low in areas where oral cancer is high.

In one study of hospitalized patients, use of vitamins C and E seemed to confer protection against esophageal cancer, and vitamin E alone or in a multivitamin supplement helped protect against oral cancer. Consuming fruits and vegetables also helped prevent oral cancer.[56]

Leukoplakia is a potentially precancerous change in the lining of the mouth. Several studies have found positive results from a supplement of beta-carotene or vitamin A.[57]

Vitamin E has also worked well in cases of leukoplakia.[58] A third antioxidant agent, NAC, a derivative of cysteine, an antioxidant amino acid (see "Cysteine"), is also promising. NAC is currently being used by EUROSCAN, a European Organization of Research and Treatment of Cancer (EORTC) in clinical trials for patients with oral or lung cancer.[59]

Ovary

Ovarian cancer is more prevalent in the Western world, which leads to the suspicion that it is diet related. Although there is little consensus on the effect of individual nutrients on the development of ovarian cancer, eating a diet rich in fruits and vegetables does seem to lower your risk.[60]

Pancreas

Smoking and a Western, high-fat diet are the two main risk factors for pancreatic cancer. Like the other cancers mentioned in this chapter, pancreatic cancer is less evident among people who eat a great deal of fruits and yellow and green vegetables.[61]

Prostate

Around 106,000 men will be diagnosed with prostate cancer within the year. It is most common in men over the age of 60, and appears to be related both to genetics and to our high-fat Western diet. There is a dramatic difference in incidence of prostate cancer between ethnic groups around the world: Prostate cancer is almost nonexistent in China, and rare in Japan. It is found among Chinese Americans and Japanese Americans, but these groups are still at lower risk than White Americans. Black men in the United States have the highest rate in the world. There is a 120-fold difference between the rate of prostate cancer for a Chinese male in Shanghai and a black male in San Francisco.[62]

Vasectomy increases a man's risk of prostate cancer by 56 percent; the longer the time since the vasectomy, the greater the risk, so after 20 years the risk of cancer rises by 86 percent above that of men without vasectomies.[63] Yet another risk is exposure to herbicides, including those used in the garden.[64]

Once again, yellow and green vegetables seem to protect men against this form of cancer.[65] Carotenes and vitamin A, particularly, have stood out as protective in some studies, though not in others.

Skin

People with light colored skin are at risk of basal cell or squamous cell cancer, especially if they spend appreciable amounts of time in the sun. Others are at risk if exposed to radium, coal tar, pitch, arsenic compounds, or creosote. Over 700,000 cases a year of these forms of skin cancer occur in the United States, and are fairly easily cured.

One man had 30 squamous cell lesions on his hands. Both

hands were going to be amputated, until he was given a derivative of vitamin A called isotretinoin (12-*cis*-retinoic acid). At the time his case was described in the medical literature, he had been free of cancer for 2 years.[66]

Preventing Basal Cell or Squamous Cell Carcinoma. In terms of prevention, wear a cover up and watch your diet! One study found lower selenium in the blood of basal or squamous cell carcinoma patients than in matched controls. People with the lowest levels of selenium had twice the risk of skin cancer as those with the highest levels.[67] Another study, in Australia, compared the diets of 80 men with basal and squamous cell carcinoma with men free of skin cancer. Eating cruciferous vegetables (brussels sprouts, broccoli, cauliflower, and cabbage), eating foods rich in vitamin C and beta-carotene (yellow, orange, and green fruits and vegetables), and eating fish protected patients from skin cancer.[68] Other studies point to bioflavonoids, which are antioxidant nutrients found along with vitamin C in fresh fruits and berries, as inhibitors of the development of squamous cell carcinoma.[69]

Recently, several studies by Chithan Kandaswami at the State University of New York at Buffalo suggest certain flavonoids, namely tangeretin, quercetin, and nobiletin, inhibited squamous cell carcinoma. The researcher found that adding flavonoids to vitamin C was a more potent inhibitor of squamous cell cancer than was vitamin C alone.[70]

Melanoma. The most dangerous kind of skin cancer is called melanoma. The incidence of this disease has risen about 4 percent per year since 1973, with about 32,000 persons diagnosed in 1993. The cause of melanoma's climbing rate is controversial. Some researchers blame artificial light, electromagnetic radiation from our consumer electrical devices and power lines, chemical additives in food that make us more sensitive to sunlight, and even sunscreen itself (because it only blocks the ultraviolet wavelengths that cause sunburn, but not the ones that pierce the skin and can initiate cancer).[71]

In an Australian study published in 1993, researchers found that women who drank two or more alcoholic drinks a day had 2.5 times the risk of malignant melanoma as nondrinkers. The study also found a diet rich with antioxidant vitamins A and E can help protect women from this dangerous form of cancer.[72]

Other studies suggest that vitamin C, vitamin A, beta-carotene, and vitamin E are particularly useful against melanoma.[73]

Stomach

In the fall of 1982, the National Research Council's Committee on Diet, Nutrition, and Cancer concluded that consumption of foods high in vitamin C is associated with a lower risk of cancers of the stomach and esophagus. One probable explanation is that vitamin C stops the transformation of the food preservatives sodium nitrite and sodium nitrate (which are widely used in packaged meats) into carcinogenic nitrosamines. For this reason, it is useful to eat tomatoes and broccoli or to drink orange juice with your hot dog or bologna sandwich!

Where salted, pickled food is used (as in the areas of the world still lacking personal refrigerators), stomach cancer is still a problem. The incidence of this form of cancer has significantly dropped in North America during the past 60 years. Thanks to safe storage capabilities, we are able to enjoy the raw fruits and vegetables and whole grains (brown rice, whole wheat, oatmeal) throughout the year and in quantities that lower our risk of stomach cancer.[74]

Urological Organs

Tobacco and diet, once again, stand out as the main risk factors for cancer of the kidney and urinary tract. A high-fat and high-protein diet seems particularly linked to kidney cancer in women, as does obesity. Excess weight contributes excess estrogen, which can imbalance pituitary hormones, and which, at least in laboratory studies, has encouraged the development of cancer.

In a 1990 Swedish study, vitamin A supplements over a 10-year period helped protect subjects from urinary tract cancer. Vitamin

C also seemed an important part of the prevention program, while fried foods and exposure to industrial chemicals increased risk.[75]

Uterus

The lining of the uterus is called the endometrium. Like breast cancer, endometrial cancer seems linked in some way to excessive exposure to the female hormone estrogen. Women at greater risk of endometrial cancer started menstruating at an early age (before age 11), experienced menopause later (after age 50), or take estrogen replacement therapy without progesterone.

Yellow and green fruits and vegetables are an important part of a dietary defense program to guard against cancer of the uterus, as well as most other cancers.[76]

Notes

1. Gao, Chang-Ming, et al. (1993). Protective effects of raw vegetables and fruit against lung cancer among smokers and ex-smokers: A case-control study in the Tokai area of Japan. *Japanese Journal of Cancer Research* 84, 594–600.
2. Ingram, Bill. (1993). The mind's supreme test—cancer. *Medical Tribune*, July 22, pp. 1, 8.
3. Laino, Charlene. (1993). With cancer rates up, environment is blamed. *Medical Tribune*, April 29, p. 1. Cited in Hamilton, Kirk. (1993). *Clinical Pearls* (p. 5). Sacramento, CA: ITServices.
4. *Cancer Facts and Figures*, 1993. American Cancer Society.
5. According to Dr. Samuel S. Epstein of the University of Illinois, although most cancer survival rates have not changed for decades, only 5% of the National Cancer Institute's $1.9 billion budget is applied to research and education on cancer prevention. The focus is instead on cancer drugs, from which pharmaceutical giants make $1 billion per year. Epstein, Samuel S. (1992). The cancer establishment. *International Journal of Health Services* 22(4), 747–749.
6. Hurley, Dan. (1992). Beta-carotene may detoxify carcinogens. *Medical Tribune*, August 20, p. 24.
7. Salmon, Andy. (1994). How does cancer begin? *California Agriculture* 48(1), 26.
8. Matanoski, Genevieve, et al. (1993). Leukemia in telephone lineman.

American Journal of Epidemiology 137(6), 609–619. Cited in Hamilton, p. 72.

9. Laino, p. 1.

10. Personal Communication, April, 1994.

11. Doll, Sir Richard. (1992). The lessons of life: Keynote address to the Nutrition and Cancer Conference. *Cancer Research* 52(Suppl.), 2024S–2029S.

12. Gao, Chang-Ming., et al. (1993). Protective effects of raw vegetables and fruit against lung cancer among smokers and ex-smokers: A case-control study in the Tokai area of Japan. *Japanese Journal of Cancer Research* 84, 594–600.

13. Kizer, Kenneth W. (1994). Public health, agriculture can forge new partnerships. *California Agriculture* 48(1), 38.

14. Block, Gladys. (1993). Micronutrients and cancer: Time for action? *Journal of the National Cancer Institute* 85(11), 846–848.

15. Block, Gladys. (1993). Micronutrients and cancer: Time for action? (editorial). *Journal of the National Cancer Institute* 85(11), 847.

16. van Poppel, Geert. (1993). Carotenoids and cancer: An update with emphasis on human intervention studies. *European Journal of Cancer* 29A(9), 1335–1344.

17. Feldman, E. B. (1993). Dietary intervention and chemoprevention— 1992 perspective. *Preventive Medicine* 22(5), 661–666. Kaizer, Leonard, et al. (1989). Fish consumption and breast cancer risk: An ecological study. *Nutrition and Cancer* 12, 61. Byers, Tim, et al. (1990). New directions: The diet–cancer link. *Patient Care* 34, 48. Doll, Sir Richard. (1990). Lifestyle: An Overview. *Cancer Detection and Prevention* 14(6), 589–594. Oniang'O, Ruth K., and Rogo, K. O. (1990). Nutrition and cancer: A review. *East African Medical Journal* 67(3), 154–161. Messina, Mark, and Barnes, Stephen. (1991). The role of soy products in reducing the risk of cancer. *Journal of the National Cancer Institute* 83(8), 541–546. Weisburger, John H. (1991). Nutritional approach to cancer prevention with emphasis on vitamins, antioxidants, and carotenoids. *American Journal of Clinical Nutrition* 53(1, Suppl.), 226S–237S.

18. Steinmetz, K. A., and Potter, J. D. (1991). Vegetables, fruit, and cancer. II. Mechanisms. *Cancer Causes and Control* 2(6), 427–242.

19. Modan, B., et al. (1981). A note on the role of dietary retinol and carotene on human gastrointestinal cancer. *British Journal of Cancer* 28, 421–424.

20. The Alpha-Tocopherol, Beta Carotene Cancer Prevention Study Group. (1994). The effect of vitamin E and beta carotene on the inci-

dence of lung cancer and other cancers in male smokers. *The New England Journal of Medicine* 330(15), 1029–1035.

21. Block, Gladys. (1991). Vitamin C and cancer prevention: the epidemiologic evidence. *American Journal of Clinical Nutrition* 53(1 Suppl.), 270S–282S.

22. Frei, Balz. (1991). Ascorbic acid protects lipids in human plasma and low-density lipoprotein against oxidative damage. *American Journal of Clinical Nutrition* 54(6), 1113S–1118S.

23. Enstrom, J. E. et al. (1992). Vitamin C intake and mortality among a sample of the United States population. *Epidemiology* 3(3), 194–202.

24. Levin, Bernard. (1992). Nutrition and colorectal cancer. Cancer, September 15, (Suppl. 70) (6), 1723–1726. Cited in Hamilton, Kirk. (1992). *Clinical Pearls* (p. 121). Sacramento, CA: ITServices.

25. Weisburger, p. 226S–237S.

26. Costa, A., et al. (1993). Retinoids and tamoxifen in breast cancer chemoprevention. *International Journal of Clinical Laboratory Research* 23(2), 53–55.

27. Levy, Louis, and Vredevoe, Donna L. (1983). The effect of N-acetylcysteine on cyclophosphamide immunoregulation and antitumor activity. *Seminars in Oncology* 10(1) (Suppl. 1), 7–16. Yarbo, John W., et al. (eds.)

28. Kim, J.A., et al. (1983). Topical use of N-acetylcysteine for reduction of skin reaction to radiation therapy. *Seminars in Oncology* 10(1), 86–88.

29. Bendich, Adrianne. (1993). Vitamin E and human immune functions. In *Human Nutrition—A Comprehensive Treatise* (Chapt. 10, pp. 217–228). Cited in Hamilton (1993), p. 183.

30. Wood, L. (1985). Possible prevention of adriamycin-induced alopecia by tocopherol. *New England Journal of Medicine* 312, 1060. Coudray, C., et al. (1992). Effects of adriamycin on chronic cardiotoxicity in selenium deficient rats. *Basic Research in Cardiology* 87, 1173–1183. Myers, C. E., et al. (1976). Adriamycin: amelioration of toxicity by alpha-tocopherol. *Cancer Treatment Report* 60, 961–962. Sonnevald, P. (1978). Effect of alpha-tocopherol on cardiotoxicity of adriamycin in the rat. *Cancer Treatment Report* 62, 1033–1036. Fujita, K., et al. Reduction of adriamycin toxicity by ascorbate in mice and guinea pig. *Cancer Research* 42, 309–316.

31. Matsukawa, Y., et al. (1993). Genistein arrests cell cycle progression at G2-M. *Cancer Research* 53, 1328–1331.

32. Ames, Bruce N. (1994). Understanding the causes of aging and cancer. *Nutrition Report* 12(6), 41,48.

33. Silverman, D. T., et al. (1992). Epidemiology of bladder cancer. *Hematology and Oncology Clinics of North America* 6(1), 1–30.

34. Laino, Charlene. (1993). Vitamins boost bladder cancer survival rates. *Medical Tribune*, June 10, p. 3.

35. Epstein, p. 47–749.

36. Ibid.

37. Hankin, J. H. (1993). Role of nutrition in women's health: diet and breast cancer. *Journal of the American Dietetic Association* 93(9), 994–999.

38. Howe, Geoffrey R., et al. (1990). Dietary factors and the risk of breast cancer: Combined analysis of 12 case-controlled studies. *Journal of the National Cancer Institute* 82, 561–569.

39. Weisburger, p. 226S–237S.

40. Hunter, D. J., *et al.* (1993). A prospective study of the intake of vitamins C, E, and A and the risk of breast cancer. *New England Journal of Medicine* 329(4), 234–240. Dajani, Esam Z. (1993). Omega-3 fatty acids and bowel cancer. *Gastroenterology* 104(4), 1238–1241.

41. Mehta, R., et al. (1985). Significance of retinol binding protein in breast tumor recurrence. *Breast Cancer* 6, 176.

42. (1990). Vitamin A used to treat cancers. *Obesity Update*, July/August, p. 8.

43. Doll, R., and Peto, R. (1981). The causes of cancer: Quantitative estimates of avoidable risks of cancer. *Journal of the National Cancer Institute* 66, 1191–1308. Burnstein, M. J. (1993). Dietary factors related to colorectal neoplasms. *Surgical Clinics of North America* 73(1), 13–29.

44. Tajima, K., et al. (1985). Urban-rural differences in the trend of colorectal cancer mortality with special reference to the subsites of colon cancer in Japan. *Gann* 76, 717–728. Cited in Weisburger, J. H. (1991). Nutritional approach to cancer prevention with emphasis on vitamins, antioxidants, and carotenoids. *American Journal of Clinical Nutrition* 53(Suppl. 1), 226S–237S.

45. Howe, G. R., et al. (1992). Dietary intake of fiber and decreased risk of cancers of the colon and rectum: Evidence from the combined analysis of 13 case-control studies. *Journal of the National Cancer Institute* 84(24), 1851–1853.

46. Giovannucci, Edward, et al. (1993). Folate, Methionine, and Alcohol Intake and Risk of Colorectal Adenoma. *Journal of the National Cancer Institute* 85(11), 875–881.

47. Bostick, R. M., et al. (1993). Reduced risk of colon cancer with high intake of vitamin E: The Iowa Women's Health Study. *Cancer Research* 53(18), 4230–4237.

48. Phillips, R., et al. (1993). Beta-carotene inhibits rectal mucosal

ornithine decarboxylase activity in colon cancer. *Cancer Research* 53, 3723–3725.

49. Huang, M. E., et al. (1988). Use of all-trans retinoic acid in the treatment of acute prolyelocytic leukemia. *Blood* 72, 567.

50. Tsutani, Hiroshi, et al. (1991). Pharmacological studies of reinol palmitate and its clinical effect in patients with acute non-lymphocytic leukemia. *Leukemia Research* 15(6), 463–471.

51. Gao, pp. 594–600.

52. Dartigues, J. F., et al. (1990). Dietary vitamin A, beta-carotene and risk of epidermoid lung cancer in southwestern France. *European Journal of Epidemiology* 6(3), 261–265.

53. Coultas, D. B., and Samet, J. M. (1992). Occupational lung cancer. *Clinics in Chest Medicine* 13(2), 341–354.

54. Menzel, Daniel B. (1992). Effect of exposure to air pollution on the need for antioxidant vitamins. *Beyond Deficiency: New Views on Function and Health Effects of Vitamins.* New York Academy of Sciences; February 9–12, Abstract 13.

55. Jaakola, K., et al. (1992). Treatment with antioxidant and other nutrients in combination with chemotherapy and irradiation in patients with small-cell lung cancer. *Anticancer Research* 12, 599–606.

56. Barone, J., Taioli, E., Hebert, J. R., and Wyndcr, E. L. (1992). Vitamin supplement use and risk for oral and esophageal cancer. *Nutrition and Cancer* 18(1), 31–41.

57. Richie, John P. (1991). Role of nutrition in cancer of the oral cavity. *Journal of Applied Nutrition* 43(1), 49–57. Garewal, Harinder S. (1992). Potential role of beta-carotene and antioxidant vitamins in the prevention of oral cancer. *Beyond Deficiency: New Views on the Function and Health Effects of Vitamins.* New York Academy of Sciences, February 9–12, p. 23.

58. Gridley, G., et al. (1992). Vitamin supplement use and reduced risk of oral and pharyngeal cancer. *American Journal of Epidemiology* 135(10), 1083–1092. Benner, S. E., et al. (1993). Regression of oral leukoplakia with alpha-tocopherol: A community clinical oncology program chemoprevention study. *Journal of the National Cancer Institute* 85(1), 44–47.

59. De Vries, N., De Flora, S. (1993). *N*-acetyl-l-cysteine. *Journal of Cell Biochemistry* 17F(Suppl.), 270–277.

60. Weisburger, p. 226S–237S.

61. Ibid.

62. (1992). Stanford Research on Prostate Cancer Aims at Lifestyle. *Geriatric Consultant*, March/April, 9.

63. Giovannucci, Edward, et al. (1993). A retrospective cohort study of vasectomy and prostate cancer in U.S. men. *Journal of the American Medical Association* 269(7), 878–882.

64. Morrison, Howard, et al. (1993). Farming and prostate cancer mortality. *American Journal of Epidemiology* 137(3), 263–269. See also Laino, p. 1.

65. Weisburger, pp. 226S–237S.

66. (1990). Vitamin A used to treat cancers. *Obesity Update*, July/August, p. 8.

67. Clark, L. C., et al. (1985). Plasma selenium and skin neoplasms: A case control study. *Nutrition and Cancer* 6, 13.

68. Kune, Gabriel A., et al. (1992). Diet, alcohol, smoking, serum beta-carotene and vitamin A in male nonmelanocytic skin cancer patients and controls. *Nutrition and Cancer* 18, 237–244.

69. Ashton, J. F., and Laura, R. S. (1993). Environmental factors and the etiology of melanoma. *Cancer Causes and Controls* 4, 59–62.

70. Kandaswami, Chithan, et al. (1993). Ascorbic acid enhanced antiproliferative effect of flavonoids on squamous cell carcinoma in vitro. *Anticancer Drugs* 4(1), 91–96. Kandaswami, Chithan, et al. (1992). Differential inhibition of proliferation of human squamous cell carcinoma, gliosarcoma and embryonic fibroblast-lung cells in culture by plant flavonoids. *Anticancer Drugs* 3(5), 525–30. Cited in Hamilton (1993), p. 82.

71. Garland, Cedric F., et al. (1993). Rising trends in melanoma: An hypothesis concerning sunscreen effectiveness. *Annals of Epidemiology* 3(1), 99–102.

72. Bain, Christopher, et al. (1993). Diet and melanoma: An exploratory case-controlled study. *Annals of Epidemiology* 3(3), 235–238.

73. Marchand, Loic Le. (1992). Dietary factors in the etiology of melanoma. *Clinics in Dermatology* 10, 79–82.

74. Hoshiyama, Yoshiharu, and Takafumi, Sasaba. (1992). A case-controlled study of stomach cancer and its relationship to diet, cigarettes and alcohol consumption and Saltama Prefecture, Japan. *Cancer Causes and Control* 3, 441–448. Weisburger (1991). Hansson, Lars-Erik, et al. (1993). Diet and risk of gastric cancer. A population-based case-control study in Sweden. *International Journal of Cancer* 55, 181–189.

75. Steineck, G., et al. (1990). Vitamin A supplements, fried foods, fat and urothelial cancer: A case-referent study in Stockholm in 1985–87. *International Journal of Cancer* 45, 1006–1011.

76. Barbone, Fabio, et al. (1993). "Diet and endometrial cancer: A case-controlled study. *American Journal of Epidemiology* 137(4), 393–403.

Cardiovascular Disease

Oxygen loves fat and oil, but turns them rancid after embracing them too long. Unfortunately, you have fat within every cell of your body, and there are times when you too turn rancid. When this damage occurs in a blood vessel, cardiovascular disease may result.

Preventing Heart Attacks and Stroke

The Greek word for heart is *kardia*, and the medical term vascular is from the Latin word *vasculum*, meaning a small vessel. Cardiovascular disease refers to abnormal conditions of both the heart itself and the veins, arteries, and capillaries that carry blood to and from the heart.

More than one in five Americans have some form of cardiovascular disease, which is the nation's number one killer. In fact, according to the American Heart Association, someone dies from cardiovascular disease every 34 seconds,[1] so finding a cure and a way to prevent its occurrence—and recurrence—is of critical importance.

Getting to the Heart of the Matter

When you think of fat you probably think of your waistline or thighs. This is a form of fat called adipose tissue, which expands

Cardiovascular Disease

What is cardiovascular disease? Cardiovascular disease refers to abnormal conditions of both the heart and the veins, arteries, and capillaries that carry blood to and from the heart.

Why is it dangerous? Blood clots or built-up plaque composed of cholesterol, blood cells, minerals, and waste can close off blood vessels. Organs affected by decreased blood can malfunction, and if the heart is affected, a heart attack can be fatal. In the brain, a blocked blood vessel can cause a debilitating or fatal stroke. Stroke and heart attack can also result from a hardening of blood vessels, called sclerosis, that makes them brittle and easily burst.

How does it happen? Plaque develops when the level of vitamins A, C, E, and beta-carotene in the blood is too low to prevent oxidation of a form of blood fat called low density lipoprotein (LDL). As a result, the LDL, in combination with certain immune cells, invades the lining of the blood vessels. At that site of invasion a build-up of body waste, minerals, blood cells, and cholesterol grows until it blocks the passage of blood through the vessel. Another explanation blames a different lipoprotein, called lipoprotein(a), as the invader that is deposited in artery walls to initiate the formation of plaque, an invasion assisted by too low a level of vitamin C and other nutrients in body cells.

Clots form when blood cells called platelets become sticky and block vessels, causing damage to the tissues behind the clot. In the brain this causes a stroke. Near the heart it can cause a heart attack.

when you eat more calories than you use up by exercise or daily living. There are other kinds of fat in your body, called triglycerides and cholesterol. These kinds of fat are floating in your bloodstream, and in scientific circles they are termed lipids

Sclerosis happens when minerals and cholesterol, a blood fat, combine along blood vessel walls to harden the walls and cause them to become so brittle they burst. If they don't burst, they can become so inflexible that blood pressure rises, and this, too, can cause a heart attack or stroke.

What can you do to protect yourself? Increase your consumption of foods rich in vitamins E and C, beta-carotene, and selenium. Vitamin E dissolves blood clots, widens the inner diameter of blood vessels, and prevents oxidation of LDL. Vitamin C protects vitamin E from being used up, prevents oxidation of LDL cholesterol, strengthens blood vessel walls, and prevents the invasion of the wall by LDL and lipoprotein(a). Beta-carotene prevents LDL from oxidation and increases HDL (high density lipoprotein), a beneficial, protective form of blood fat. Selenium is needed for the activity of an important antioxidant enzyme called glutathione peroxidase, which removes dangerous oxidants from the blood.

What additional nutrients are needed? The following nutrients are also needed: magnesium (a deficiency enhances atherosclerosis), omega-3 fatty acids (adequately provided by two high-fat fish meals per week, such as salmon, anchovies, herring, and sardines), flavonoids (to strengthen vessel walls and inhibit oxidation of LDL. Flavonoids are found in the white rind of citrus fruit; in other fruits and vegetables, particularly apples and onions; and in red wine and tea), Ginkgo biloba (the leaves of this ornamental tree increase blood flow in the brain, fight free radicals, and prevent lipid peroxidation), and garlic (reduces triglycerides and cholesterol, reduces blood pressure, and reduces the formation of clots).

Blood is a watery solution. Fat and water don't easily mix, so any fat-soluble substance, be it triglycerides, cholesterol, or vitamins A or E, must have a companion along to keep it soluble in blood. Lipids are transported through the blood on protein-coated companions called lipoproteins.

The official story of cardiovascular disease begins with lipoproteins. The cholesterol in our blood is composed of two kinds of lipoproteins: high density lipoproteins (HDL) and low density lipoproteins (LDL).

Normal LDL molecules contain vitamin E, beta-carotene, and another carotene called lycopene. As long as these three nutrients are present, normal LDL cannot be damaged by oxidation.[2]

When body stores of antioxidants are low, oxidation of LDL occurs. Apparently, specialized immune cells called monocytes are particularly attracted to oxidized LDL. Especially if there is some copper or iron in the blood, the monocytes cling to the oxidized LDL and together they invade the lining of the blood vessel. Inside the vessel wall, the monocytes transform into a new kind of immune cell, called a macrophage, which further oxidizes the LDL and forms yet another entity, called a *foam cell*. The foam cells add to the damage of the blood vessel wall and cause a fatty streak[3] (see Figure 2).

By itself, a fatty streak is not dangerous. However, foam cells become part of a deteriorating situation in the artery wall and dietary fats, calcium, blood cells, and body trash that normally would be absorbed into the intestines clump together at the site of damage, like a pileup on a busy freeway. This collection of rubbish hardens over time into an immovable mass that keeps grow-

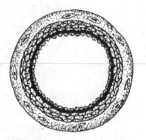 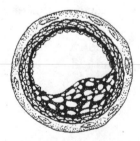

Figure 2 Cross-section of (*left*) a clean, healthy artery and (*right*) an artery showing infiltration of fat in the inner wall.

ing as more debris accumulates. What began as a little damaged area turns into a major impediment to blood flow. Slowly, over months and years, the opening in the blood vessel narrows without any outward sign of it happening, until, if the damaged area is in an artery leading to the heart, the vessel becomes so closed off it can no longer provide enough blood to keep the heart functioning. That's why all too often the first sign of cardiovascular disease is death from a heart attack.

Lipoprotein(a) and Vitamin C

For a number of years, scientists have noted the existence of a form of lipoprotein other than LDL, called lipoprotein(a). Some researchers, including the late Linus Pauling and others at the Linus Pauling Institute of Science and Medicine in Palo Alto, believe the deposition of lipoprotein(a) initiates plaque formation.[4]

In March 1992, Pauling announced that he and Matthias Rath, who was then director of cardiology research at the Pauling Institute, discovered a "clear connection" between lipoprotein(a) and vitamin C. According to Pauling, "Low intake of vitamin C is the primary cause of heart disease."[5] The then-nonagenarian Nobel Laureate also stated the Institute had found ways to prevent and even reverse plaque formation and angina pectoris by the use of vitamin C and other natural substances.

Whether the cause is lipoprotein(a) or LDL cholesterol, there is general agreement that antioxidants appear to beneficially influence cardiovascular disease.

White Bread and Sugar: Double Jeopardy

Why is cardiovascular disease an epidemic in America today? Two far-reaching changes in our lifestyle as compared to that of our grandparents are possibly the culprit. The first and most important is the stripping of the nutritious germ from whole wheat in the milling process. This began in 1910 and gave rise to an American love affair with white flour and white bread. When the darker colored germ was removed, a major source of vitamin E was swept away.

The second change is the incredible rise in consumption of sugar, particularly since World War II. Talk about a real love affair! Sugar is 20 percent of the diet of many Americans. In fact, white sugar is the third most frequently consumed "food" in the United States, after coffee and white bread![6]

While you can find articles in the medical literature exonerating sugar of any role in cardiovascular disease, it does increase blood uric acid and glucose levels, create red blood cell abnormalities, and lower HDL levels in the blood.[7] Some research suggests that prolonged exposure of LDL to high concentrations of glucose contributes to foam cell formation.[8]

Thus, just as Americans reduced their consumption of an excellent source of the very vitamin that protects LDL cholesterol from being oxidized and their blood vessels from being damaged, they also increased their consumption of a substance that accelerates the damage. On top of these changes, Americans stopped eating fresh fruits and vegetables as much as in generations past.

Vitamin E to the Rescue

It is too late for Dr. James Shute and his sons, Drs. Wilfrid and Evan Shute, to receive our appreciation as they've now passed on, but this family of Canadian physicians must be credited with bringing the heart healing properties of vitamin E to the attention of the world during the middle of this century.

The Shutes' early work focused on obstetrical problems, since both James and Evan were obstetrician–gynecologists. Eventually, the vitamin was given to a man in severe congestive heart failure, and his heart attack symptoms disappeared. Wilfrid, the family cardiologist, then entered the picture and began using vitamin E for heart conditions.

By 1969, when Wilfrid Shute coauthored *Vitamin E for Ailing and Healthy Hearts*, he and his staff at The Shute Institute in Pt. Credit, Ontario, had treated more than 30,000 people with cardiovascular complaints. Shute wrote: "Not only is alpha tocopherol the drug of choice in treating coronary artery narrowing and/or occlusion, but it is also effective in treating all other forms of heart disease with or without the help of other old and new drugs."[9] Shute cautions, however, that those who want to reproduce his results must carefully follow the same dosage schedule that his clinic developed.

The Right Dose. According to Shute, the correct dosage can mean the difference between success and failure—even life and death. "Different forms of cardiovascular disease require different ranges of effective dosage," Shute explains.[10] When too little blood is passing through the coronary arteries, 800 to 1,200 IU daily may be needed, though some patients may need much more. Yet, a patient with chronic rheumatic heart disease cannot tolerate such high doses, says Shute, and ought to be given no more than 90 IU daily for the first 4 weeks, increasing up to a maximum of only 150 IU. In contrast, for intermittent claudication (painful closure of blood vessels in the legs during exercise), 1,600 to 2,400 IU may be the correct dose. According to the experience of the Shutes, the correct dose is best achieved slowly, and is that which leads to improvement within 4 to 6 weeks.

Exciting New Research on Vitamin E. Long before it was fashionable to study free radical scavengers, the Shutes wrote that vitamin E's power lay not only in its ability to both widen the opening of the blood vessels and break up clots, but that it also served in the blood as an antioxidant. Vitamin E, they wrote, bonded with the polyunsaturated fatty acids released in the bloodstream by dietary fats and prevented their oxidation. However, the Shutes published during a time when nutritional solutions to medical problems were belittled and ignored. The Shutes were too enthusiastic about vitamin E therapy and too public to be considered in good taste by the medical community. Although by 1952 there were nearly four dozen published scientific studies showing positive results for cardiovascular problems using vitamin E, that same year the College of Physicians and Surgeons in Ontario Province concluded vitamin E had no place in the treatment of cardiovascular disease. And it wasn't only the Canadian medical profession which rose against tocopherol and the Shutes.

Dr. Jonathan Wright, in his April 1993 *Let's Live* magazine column, describes how a group of patients organized themselves into the Cardiac Society to publicize the Shute's successful work and attempted to sell the doctor's book as well as vitamin E capsules (which weren't generally available at the time) from an office in Detroit. According to Wright, the American Medical Association convinced the United States Postal Service to return letters addressed to the Society stamped FRAUDULENT.

Luckily for the blood vessels of North Americans, more recent research once again spotlights vitamin E as a lifesaver, and this time the vitamin's powers are not being reviled or ignored.

In Europe, for example, random samples of 100 apparently healthy men between the ages of 40 and 49 were taken from 16 large populations with widely varying death rates for heart disease. The levels of vitamin E in the blood of these men was the most important risk factor discovered, even beyond smoking. Vitamin A was a close second. In fact, the level of vitamins E and A in the blood could lead the researchers to predict 73 percent of the time which men would die from a heart attack![11]

It appears that vitamin E prevents the oxidation of LDL cholesterol,[12] increases levels of HDL cholesterol (the beneficial form of blood fat), and prevents the clumping of platelets (red blood cells) that might cause a blood clot and heart attack or stroke.

So, what happens when people take a supplement of vitamin E? In 1993, two studies from Harvard University were published that were really worth getting excited about. Over 87,000 nurses participated in the first study, which began in 1980 and included questionnaires about diet and supplement habits. Although the nurses recruited for the study considered themselves healthy, during the next 8 years some suffered heart attacks. Meir Stampfer and his colleagues found that those nurses who had reported taking at least 100 IU of vitamin E per day for at least 2 years were about 40 percent less likely to have had a heart attack than those taking less vitamin E.[13]

This study was unsettling, to say the least. Few of the nurses in the Stampfer study were obtaining any more than 8 IU of the vitamin in their diet. Yet the standard medical opinion was that the vast majority of people could obtain all the nutrients they needed directly from their meals. Then along came Stampfer's research, which clearly pointed to nutritional supplementation of vitamin E as important for protection against the oxidation of LDL cholesterol. The researchers, in fact, concluded that "supplementation at levels far higher than those achievable by diet alone may be needed to reduce LDL oxidation."

When Eric Rimm and his team waited just 4 years to document what happened to almost 40,000 male health professionals, they found quite similar results. The men who took from 100 IU to 249 IU of vitamin E a day for 2 years or more enjoyed a 37 percent lower risk of heart attack than those who didn't take supplemental E. Contrary to the "more is necessarily better" philosophy, those who supplemented even more than 249 IU a day derived no greater benefit than those taking 100 IU.[14]

There are two other major clinical trials of vitamins A, C, and E, and their effect on cardiovascular health going on right now. The results of one are due in 1998, and the other in 1999. One final word about these trials. The Stampfer and Rimm results do not indicate that nature made a mistake with us and that we are innately deficient in enough vitamin E to protect our blood vessels! Plenty of native cultures around the world, including our very own before this century, have had no problem with cardiovascular disease. The blame lies with our daily diet, not our genes. Consequently, if you aren't willing to change your diet, you'd better consider substituting in capsule form for what you're missing on your plate.

And in This Corner—Vitamin C

Over 50 years ago, a Canadian cardiologist named Patterson noticed that the vast majority of his heart disease patients were low in vitamin C. More currently, Dr. Joel Simon of the Veteran's Administration Center in San Francisco reviewed vitamin C's connection to cardiovascular disease and came up with quite a number of plausible links. For example, vitamin C prevents lipid peroxidation, particularly of LDL cholesterol; it is a major antioxidant in the watery medium of the blood; and it regenerates vitamin E.

Linus Pauling, who championed vitamin C for a quarter of a

century, described C's ability to strengthen and maintain the integrity of blood vessel walls. According to Pauling, the development of atherosclerosis is a direct result of vitamin C deficiency, since the body's build-up of plaque is its way of attempting to strengthen blood vessel walls grown weak and fragile from a lack of vitamin C.[15]

Others have documented vitamin C's ability to reduce blood pressure and raise HDL cholesterol levels, which both can help prevent heart disease.[16] As an example of vitamin C's ability to control cholesterol levels, when a group of healthy volunteers were followed for 1 year and a group of patients with vascular disease were followed for nearly 2 years, researchers found the greater the level of vitamin C in the subjects' immune cells, the lower their cholesterol levels. These researchers also noted a seasonal variation of vitamin C: ascorbate levels rose in summer and dropped in winter. However, if supplementation stopped in summer months, cholesterol rose to winter levels. "Given these findings," wrote the study authors, "we suggest that patients with vascular disease should have vitamin C supplements throughout the year."[17]

Selenium

Half a century ago, children and young women in a certain swath from southwestern to northeastern China suffered from a hardening and destruction of the heart muscle that caused many deaths. The area was called the Keshan belt. After much investigation, researchers concluded that in addition to viruses and toxins weakening the population, there was a significant deficiency of selenium in the soil. Since people in China eat locally grown food, there was therefore a deficiency of selenium in the blood of the victims. And it was this selenium deficiency that caused what became known as Keshan's disease. Today, the population of this area stays well by taking selenium supplements.

In the United States, the selenium content of the soil varies widely, but the only cases of Keshan's disease that have appeared did so in patients given long-term intravenous feeding of a solution that lacked selenium. That doesn't mean American heart attack patients have appropriate selenium. "A pattern of low selenium is often found in patients with acute myocardial infarction and in those with coronary heart disease," one study concluded in a review of selenium's role in cardiovascular disease.[18]

Selenium is essential for the optimum function of an important enzyme called glutathione peroxidase. Glutathione peroxidase protects the heart, along with the lung, liver, and blood cells, from free radical damage by transforming more highly toxic oxidants into a less toxic oxidant called hydrogen peroxide. Another enzyme, called catalase, then comes along and converts the hydrogen peroxide into harmless water and oxygen.[19]

Selenium is also antagonistic to heavy metals like cadmium, mercury, and lead, which in high doses can cause hypertension. The selenium pulls these metals out of circulation in the blood.

Flavonoids and Fatty Acids

Bioflavonoids are found in citrus fruits as well as in apples, onions, and tea.[20] Research at the National Institute of Public Health and Environmental Protection in The Netherlands looked at bioflavonoid consumption among a group of 805 men 65 to 84 years old, during a 5-year period. Those men with higher intake had lower incidence of fatal heart disease, and the link remained significant after adjustment for smoking, blood pressure, and other variables. The researchers noted that bioflavonoids are excellent free radical scavengers, which might account for the men's protection against heart attack.[21] Bioflavonoids are also famous for strengthening the walls of capillaries and other blood vessels, which certainly helps maintain a healthy cardiovascular system.

Poly Want a Phenol?

Tea is one of the most common sources of polyphenols in the average Western diet. Polyphenols stop lipid peroxidation in the membrane of red blood cells; reduce blood coagulation; increase the break-up of clots; prevent the aggregation and sticking together of red blood cells; and decrease the cholesterol content in the wall of the aorta, the body's primary artery leading from the heart. In these ways, tea helps preserve and protect the health of the cardiovascular system.[22]

A Norwegian study published in 1992 found some beneficial effects of tea drinking on cholesterol levels, particularly in people drinking five or more cups of tea a day. Systolic blood pressure and death from heart disease were both less among those drinking tea.[23] A Japanese study also suggested that drinking green tea helped lower serum cholesterol. Mean cholesterol concentrations were lower in men drinking 9 cups or more per day of green tea than they were in those consuming 0 to 2 cups per day. There was no noticeable effect on triglycerides or low density lipoproteins (LDL cholesterol).[24]

Coenzyme Q10

At the Seventh International Symposium on the Medical and Clinical Aspects of Coenzyme Q10 held in 1992, Professor Karl Folkers of the Institute for Biomedical Research, University of Texas at Austin, described several studies showing a deficiency of CoQ10 among congestive heart failure patients. Although it is common to be deficient in more than one nutrient, there seems to be a particular relationship between heart failure and the deficiency of CoQ10.

Supplementation in cases of heart failure can be of significant benefit in terms of overall health and of survival among heart surgery patients, claims Folkers. He reports the results of one study where patients were given 100 mg of CoQ10 for 2 weeks prior to heart surgery and for 30 days following surgery. Recovery time was quicker and less complicated in those patients supplemented with CoQ10 versus the controls (3 to 5 days versus 15 to 30 days, respectively).[25]

While the previous study worked with only 10 heart patients, a study in Italy looked at 2,500 patients diagnosed with heart failure described as classes II and III according to the guidelines established by the New York Heart Association. Participants took from 50 to 150 mg per day (the majority took 100 mg per day). Preliminary results are coming in and show a low incidence of side effects and a strong response: After 3 months of treatment with CoQ10, 81 percent of the patients suffered less cyanosis (turning bluish from lack of oxygen), 76.9 percent reduced their edema, 78.4 percent reduced their pulmonary rates, 82.4 percent reduced their sweating, 60.2 percent were complaining less about insomnia, 75.7 percent had less palpitations, and 73 percent had less vertigo (dizziness).[26]

In another study, 18 patients taken off all hypertension medication for 2 weeks were given either coenzyme Q10 or a placebo for 10 weeks, and after a 2-week break, the substances were switched for another 10 weeks. The CoQ10 lowered systolic blood pressure about 10 points, and the diastolic about 7 points, while the placebo group maintained the same blood pressure throughout the trial.[27]

Garlic

Garlic is a hard-working herb of great benefit for the cardiovascular system (see chapter entitled "Garlic"). Allicin, its active ingredient, is a good antioxidant and helps prevent oxidation of lipoproteins. It stops the infiltration of lipids into blood vessel walls, improves circulation of blood, lowers LDL cholesterol, reduces blood pressure, increases HDL cholesterol, and helps prevent clots.[28] Fortunately for your friends and fellow workers, there are deodorized garlic products on the market that do all the above and allow you to be sociable as well.

Ginkgo

Another herbal antioxidant useful for cardiovascular protection is the leaf of an ornamental tree called *Ginkgo biloba*. Drs. Jos Kleijnen and Paul Knipschild of The Netherlands reviewed 40 clinical trials using this herb and found only 8 among them that the two researchers considered to be well-designed and well-performed. Nevertheless, they still concluded that if they themselves suffered a lack of blood to the brain ("cerebral insufficiency") they'd take Ginkgo biloba, since there were apparently no negative side effects and every study reported positive results.[29] (See the chapter entitled "Ginkgo Biloba" for more on this herb.)

There's More to Cardio-Fitness Than Antioxidants

The first step to having a healthy heart is not the purchase of a supplement. All the substances that I have discussed thus far are secondary to exercising regularly, maintaining a healthy body weight, eating a low-fat diet, and stopping smoking. If you haven't yet invested in yourself in these important ways, start now! An excellent and amusing guide is *Dr. Dean Ornish's Program for Reversing Heart Disease*, written by San Francisco area heart health expert Dean Ornish.[30]

In addition, certain substances other than antioxidants contribute to a healthy cardiovascular system. For example, two members of the vitamin B complex, vitamin B-12 and folic acid, regulate production of an amino acid called homocysteine; a low level of homocysteine in the blood is one of the clearest signs of cardiovascular risk.[31] Another important marker of heart health is your level of blood magnesium, a mineral linked by recent scientific research to preventing heart attacks.[32]

Summary

If you'd like to keep your heart and arteries whistle clean, here are a few suggestions:

- Invest time in physical fitness. All-out effort on weekends is not healthy, but even 20 minutes several times during the week is.

- Cut the amount of fat you eat to rock bottom.

- Use frozen fruit concentrate in recipes instead of sugar.

- Plan your daily menus around whole grains (100 percent whole wheat, millet, oats, etc.), fruit, and vegetables. Keep whole wheat flour in the freezer to protect it from oxidation. Consume at least five, and preferably nine, fruits and vegetables each day.

- Look for ways to increase the variety of vegetables and fruits you consume, such as juicing them (there are several excellent juicing recipe books available) or using them in baked goods (have you ever tasted sweet potato pie or zucchini muffins? Yum!).

* Make time for pleasure. What's the use of a long life without fun?

Daily Dosage

The following dosages are recommended:

Green or black tea	5 cups
Garlic	3 capsules or 1 clove
Ginkgo biloba	120–240 mg
Vitamin C	1–3 grams
Bioflavonoids	1 gram
Vitamin E	100 IU
Selenium	50 mcg

Notes

1. American Heart Association. (1994). *Heart and Stroke Facts: 1994 Statistical Supplement.*
2. Steinberg, Daniel, et al. (1989). Beyond cholesterol: Modifications of low-density lipoprotein that increase its atherogenicity. *The New England Journal of Medicine* 320(14), 915–924.
3. Ibid.
4. Pauling, Linus. (1992). Prevention and treatment of heart disease, new research focus at the Linus Pauling Institute. Linus Pauling Institute of Science and Medicine Newsletter, March, 1.
5. Ibid.
6. Feuer, Janice. (1993). *Fruit-Sweet and Sugar-Free* (p. 6). Rochester, VT: Healing Arts Press.
7. Lithell, H., *et al.* (1985). Muscle lipoprotein lipase inactivated by ordinary amounts of dietary carbohydrates. *Human Nutrition Clinical Nutrition* 39C(4), 289–295.
8. Steinberg, p. 920.
9. Shute, Wilfrid E., with Taub, Harald J. (1969). *Vitamin E for Ailing and Healthy Hearts* (p. 176). New York: Pyramid House.

10. Ibid., p. 177.

11. Gey, K. F., et al. (1989). Inverse correlation between plasma vitamin E and mortality from ischemic heart disease in cross-cultural epidemiology. *ACTA Cardiologica* 44(6), 493–494.

12. Ferns, Gordon A. A. (1993). *Vitamin E: The evidence for an anti-atherogenic role Artery* 20(2), 61–94. Cited in Hamilton, Kirk. (1993). *Clinical Pearls* (p. 38). Sacramento, CA: ITServices.

13. Stampfer, Meir J., et al. (1993). Vitamin E consumption and the risk of coronary disease in women. *The New England Journal of Medicine* 328(20), 1444–1449.

14. Rimm, Eric B., et al. (1993). Vitamin E consumption and the risk of coronary heart disease in men *New England Journal of Medicine* 328, 1450–1456.

15. Anonymous. (1992). How vitamin C can prevent heart attack and stroke. *Linus Pauling Institute for Science and Medicine Newsletter*, March, p. 3.

16. Jacques, P. F. (1990). Effects of vitamin C on HDL and blood pressure. *Journal of the American College of Nutrition* 9(5), 554/Abstract 106.

17. MacRury, S. M., et al. (1992). Seasonal and climatic variation in cholesterol and vitamin C: Effect of vitamin C supplementation. *Scottish Medical Journal* 37(2), 49–52.

18. Oster, O., and Prellwitz, W. (1990). Selenium in cardiovascular disease. *Biological Trace Elements* 124, 91–103.

19. Bland, Jeffrey. (1986). The nutritional effects of free radical pathology. In *1986—A Year in Nutritional Medicine* (p. 304). New Canaan, CT: Keats.

20. Hertog, M., et al. (1993). Intake of potentially anticarcinogenic flavonoids and their determinants in adults in The Netherlands. *Nutrition and Cancer* 20, 21–29.

21. Hertog, M., et al. (1993). Dietary antioxidant flavonoids and risk of coronary heart disease: The Zutphen elderly study. *Lancet* 342, 1007–1011.

22. Lou, Fu-Qing, et al. (1992). A study on tea pigment in the prevention of atherosclerosis. *Preventive Medicine* 21(3), 333.

23. Stensvold, Inger, et al. (1992). Tea consumption, relationship to cholesterol, blood pressure and coronary and total mortality. *Preventive Medicine* 21, 546–553. Cited in Hamilton, Kirk. (1992). *Clinical Pearls* (p. 165). Sacramento, CA: ITServices.

24. Kono, Suminori, et al. (1992). Green tea consumption and serum lipid profiles: A cross-sectional study in northern Kyushu, Japan. *Preventive Medicine* 21, 526–531. Cited in Hamilton (1992), p. 179.

25. Folkers, Karl. (1993). Heart failure as a dominant deficiency of coenzyme Q10 and challenges for future clinical research on coenzyme Q10. *Clinical Investigator* 71, S551–S554. Judy, W. V., et al. (1993). Myocardial preservation by therapy with coenzyme Q10 during heart surgery. *Clinical Investigator* 71, S155–S161. Both cited in Hamilton (1993), p. 90.

26. Baggio, E., et al. (1993). Italian multicenter study on the safety of efficiency of coenzyme Q10 as adjunctive therapy in heart failure (interim analysis). *Clinical Investigator* 71, S145–S149. Cited in Hamilton (1993).

27. Digiesi, V., et al. (1990). Effect of coenzyme Q10 on essential arterial hypertension. *Current Therapeutic Research* 47(5), 841–845.

28. Fogarty, M. (1993). Garlic's potential role in reducing heart disease. *British Journal of Clinical Practice* 47(2), 64–65.

29. Kleijnen, Jos, and Knipschild, Paul. (1992). Ginkgo biloba for cerebral insufficiency. *British Journal of Clinical Pharmacology* 34, 352–358.

30 Ornish, Dean. (1990). *Dr. Dean Ornish's Program for Reversing Heart Disease*. New York, Ballantine Books.

31. Olszewski, Andrzej J., and McCully, Kilmer S. (1993). Homocysteine metabolism and the oxidative modification of proteins and lipids. *Free Radical Biology and Medicine* 14, 683–693. Cited in Hamilton (1993), p. 35.

32. Millane, T. A., and Camm, A. J. (1992). Magnesium and the myocardium. *British Heart Journal* 68, 441–442. Cited in Hamilton (1993), p. 93.

~~~ Cataracts

If you could peek inside the pupil of your own eye, you'd see a small clear disk hanging just beyond the opening, suspended by delicate fibers. This is the crystalline lens. It is responsible for focusing light onto the retina, a specialized area at the back of your eyeball. By adjusting light onto the retina, the lens ensures the image remains sharply in focus whether it is nearby or far away. The retina then sends the light image as a message up the optic nerve to the brain and you "see" the image. As you age, proteins damaged by free radicals accumulate, lump together, precipitate out, and fog the formerly clear lens. This fogging of the lens is called a cataract.

In the United States, over 2 million people suffer from cataracts. In fact, they occur in as many as 46 percent of people over the age of 75. Fifty million people worldwide are blind because of cataracts. In North America, surgery and replacement lenses are the rule, and blindness is unusual. However, cataract removal surgery and related office visits require the largest proportion of the Medicare budget, adding up to more than $3 billion annually. The search for a way to prevent cataracts is fueled by the knowledge that if cataract formation were delayed by even 5 years, half the surgeries now performed would not be needed.

When you look at a map of the world superimposed on a map of cataract occurrence, it is apparent that cataracts are most problematic where sunlight is most intense and long lasting. Ultraviolet light is known to create free radicals, which are a common cause of the damage that fogs our lenses. However, even something as unchangeable as sunlight doesn't have to give you cataracts, if you protect yourself by consuming nutritional antioxidants.[1] For example, there is evidence that adequate doses of beta-carotene and vitamin B-2 (riboflavin) can help prevent the formation of cataracts.

When patients with cataracts are asked about their diet, researchers find they are less likely to eat enough foods rich in vitamins A, C, or E, and less likely to take supplements of vitamins E or C.[2] People with diabetes, who are highly at risk for cataracts and other eye problems, might want to make sure their diets are rich with these antioxidants well before they enter their later years.

Beta-Carotene

Beta-carotene is one of the the most important nutrients related to cataract prevention. For example, University of Illinois at Chicago researchers injected rats with beta-carotene, then exposed their eyes to light. The injected rats suffered less eye damage than did unexposed rats.[3]

Vitamin C

Of all body sites, the eye has the highest levels of vitamin C. This suggests that vitamin C may be used to protect against oxidative damage from heat and ultraviolet radiation, as well as to promote wound healing in the eye.[4] Interestingly, animals that are active at night do not have nearly as much vitamin C in their eyes as animals active in the daytime. This makes sense because of vitamin C's role in protecting the eye from damage by ultraviolet light, which is strongest during the day.

Our eyes accumulate about 20 to 70 times the amount of vitamin C found in the blood. Vitamin C plays many roles in eye health. For example, it is involved in the metabolism of fat and iron, it stimulates hormones, and it helps synthesize proteins. The role we are most interested in is its use as an antioxidant, which it does nobly in two ways. First, vitamin C helps us eliminate oxygen from the lens, reducing the possibility of damage from ultraviolet-light-induced free radicals that produce cataracts. Second, it helps vitamin E return to active duty as vitamin E is used up.

In 1993, Allen Taylor and his colleagues at the Laboratory for Nutrition and Vision Research at Tufts University revealed the results of their research comparing cataract development among people who consumed lots of antioxidants and those who didn't consume the nutrients. People in their study who consumed over 300 mg of vitamin C a day had a third the risk of developing cataracts as people who consumed less vitamin C.

Bioflavonoids

Bioflavonoids are found in nature along with vitamin C, mostly in the white inner rind of citrus fruits. There are a number of bioflavonoids, and one, called *rutin*, has been linked with cataract prevention.

When animals are fed a lot of sugar, an enzyme in the eye called *aldose reductase* changes the sugar molecules into a form of alcohol that accumulates over time and causes the lens to swell and fibers in the lens to rupture, leading to cataract.[5] Bioflavonoids prevent formation of the enzyme, and help protect the lens from damage.

Vitamin E

In the Taylor study at Tufts mentioned under vitamin C, the researchers also found those taking 400 IU of vitamin E per day had a third the risk of developing cataracts as those taking less vitamin E. In another study, researchers at the Dana Center for Preventive Ophthalmology (Wilmer Eye Institute) at Johns Hopkins Medical Institutions in Baltimore found that people who developed cataracts had lower levels of vitamin E in their blood than those who didn't develop the condition.[6]

Selenium

Several studies have reported a connection between a diet low in selenium and the appearance of opaque lenses, particularly in laboratory animals. Since selenium works synergistically with vitamin E and all the antioxidants seem to work best in unison, a comprehensive cataract-prevention formula should include selenium.

Bilberry

In 1989, researchers tested bilberry's effectiveness in cases of cataract. They gave both vitamin E and bilberry to 50 elderly people for 4 months. Cataracts stopped developing in 97 percent of the subjects![7]

L-Cysteine and L-Methionine

L-Cysteine and L-methionine are amino acids that are potent antioxidants useful in the treatment of cataracts. Both are critical in the creation of the enzyme glutathione, which protects the lens from ultraviolet light. With age, the amount of glutathione available diminishes. Supplementing with L-cysteine and L-methionine is thought to retard this decline in glutathione and thereby help prevent the cataracts that result from ultraviolet light damage.[8]

Treating Existing Cataracts

Most of the research published in the medical literature is on preventing cataracts, not treating existing opacities. One study found improved vision from 4 to 8 weeks after patients began taking 350 mg of vitamin C daily among 60 percent of patients with beginning signs of cataract. Unfortunately, patients with preexisting cataracts were not affected by this level of supplementation.[9]

This doesn't mean reversal can't happen. It means a nutritional reversal method for people hasn't yet been perfected. There is, for example, a report in the medical literature of mature cataracts in dogs clearing 72 hours after being injected with superoxide dismutase (SOD), an enzyme that destroys the superoxide free radical. This technique is not yet performed on human beings.[10]

Prevention

George Bunce of the Virginia Polytechnic Institute advises us to take 200 to 400 IU of vitamin E and 100 to 250 mg of vitamin C daily, in addition to eating a diet rich in fruits and vegetables. "I take the position that these daily supplements are unlikely to be injurious and are likely to confer a beneficial level of resistance against unavoidable oxidant stress in many tissues of the body, including the eye," writes Bunce in a recent article in the *Journal of Nutritional Biochemistry*.[11] As evident from the supplement recommendations elsewhere in this book, Bunce's recommendations for vitamin C are modest, though he insists they assure a saturation of your tissues at a safe level.

While it is possible to reverse cataracts in their earliest stages, it is always easier to prevent the development of this condition than to treat already existing cataracts. With a proper diet and supplement program, as many as a third of cataracts can be prevented.[12]

Daily Dosage

Vitamin A	5,000 to 10,000 IU
Beta-carotene	5,000 IU
Vitamin C	250 mg or to bowel tolerance
Vitamin E	600 to 800 IU
Selenium	400 mcg
Bilberry	300 mg
L-Cysteine	400 mg

Notes

1. Varma, S. D. (1991). Scientific basis for medical therapy of cataracts by antioxidants. *American Journal of Clinical Nutrition* 53(1, Suppl.), 335S–345S. See also errata published in 55(1), iv.

2. Garland, D. (1991). Ascorbic acid and the eye. *American Journal of Clinical Nutrition* 54, 1198S–1202S8. See also Mohan, Madan, et al. (1989). India–U.S. case-control study of age-related cataracts. *Archives of Ophthalmology* 107(5), 670–676.

3. Bunce, George E. (1979). Nutrition and cataract. *Nutrition Reviews* 37(11), 337–343.

4. Garland, pp. 670–676.

5. Bland, Jeffrey. (1991). *Delicious!* May/June, 14–15.

6. Vitale, S., et al. (1993). Plasma antioxidants and risk of cortical and nuclear cataract. *Epidemiology* 4(3), 195–203.

7. Bravetti, et al. (1989). *Annali di Ottalmologia and Clinica Oculistica* 15, 109. Cited in Schechter, Steven R. (1994). Herbs for life—Bilberry extract: Nature's circulatory, visionary aid. *Let's Live*, March, 70.

8. Garner, M. H., and Spector, A. (1980). Selective oxidation of cysteine and methionine in normal and senile cataractous lenses. *Proceedings of the National Academy of Sciences*, USA 77(3), 1274–1277. See also Cole, H. (1985). Enzyme activity may hold the key to cataract activity. *Journal of the American Medical Association* 254(8), 1008. Both cited in Werbach, Melvyn R. (1993). Cataract. *Nutritional Influences on Illness, Second Edition* (p. 201). Tarzana, CA: Third Line Press.

9. Bouton, S. M., Jr. (1939). Vitamin C and the aging eye. *Archives of Internal Medicine* 63, 930–945.

10. Lynd, F. T., and McDonald, N. (1978). The treatment of senile cataracts in dogs by the intra-ocular injection of superoxide dismutase. *Journal of Veterinary Pharmacology and Therapy* 1, 85–88.

11. Bunce, G. E. (1994). Nutrition and eye disease of the elderly. *Journal of Nutritional Biochemistry* 5, 66–77.

12. Bunce, G. E., personal communication, September 19, 1994.

Exercise-Induced Free Radical Damage

If exercise could be packed into a pill, it would be the single most widely prescribed, and beneficial, medicine in the nation.

—Robert Butler, former director
National Institute on Aging

Few would argue that regular exercise is an important part of a health maintenance program. Whether you are young or old, exercise improves your muscle tone, reduces your risk of heart disease[1] and cancer,[2] reduces cholesterol, keeps your bones strong, thickens your skin to prevent sagging,[3] helps you sleep better, controls your weight, improves your self-esteem,[4] increases the activity of a virus-fighting protein called interferon,[5] and is a useful tonic for depression.[6] Scientists agree that exercise sessions ranging from three sessions of 30 minutes of exercise per week up to 1 hour every day will alter your biochemistry in beneficial ways.[7]

What you may not have read is how exercise alters your biochemistry in non-beneficial ways, specifically by the creation of free radicals, which contribute to muscle damage. For example, investigators from Rowett Research Institute, Bucksburn, and the University Medical School (both located in Aberdeen, United Kingdom) measured oxidative stress in runners by comparing blood samples before and after exercise. Their results show that muscle damage occurs when even trained athletes run a comparatively short distance, and red blood cells are at least temporarily more susceptible to peroxidation.[8] Thus, it isn't surprising that studies at Washington University School of Medicine (St. Louis), the Technion-Israel Institute of Technology, and elsewhere show that supplemental antioxidant vitamins offer a definite improvement in the body's defense against these free radicals and better recovery of the muscles after vigorous exercise.[9]

A deficiency of vitamin E increases the oxidation of fats (a process called lipid peroxidation), decreases the soundness of cell membranes, and reduces the ability of the body to use oxygen. Should athletes take vitamin E to improve performance? You will find ardent opinions in both camps.

Thomas Cureton conducted 42 experiments involving nearly 900 human subjects at the University of Illinois from 1950 to 1969, in which he compared the endurance, physical fitness, speed of recovery from oxygen debt, and other physiological parameters between those taking wheat germ oil (a potent source of vitamin E) and those taking a variety of placebos. His results, published in 1972,[10] emphasized the benefit of a component of wheat germ oil called octacosanol in improving the endurance of his subjects. However, attempts to replicate his findings have been inconsistent. Some researchers found benefit of octacosanol, but others found none.[11]

Vitamin E supplementation seems of particular benefit to athletic endeavors at high altitudes,[12] but not such a significant help at sea level.[13] Nevertheless, because of the known benefits of antioxidant vitamins C and E on connective tissue and muscle recovery, it is expected that supplementation of these nutrients will be of benefit to any exerciser, be they in athletes scaling mountains or weekend walkers.[14]

Coenzyme Q10 (CoQ10) is another important nutrient for serious exercisers.[15] It is found in greatest concentration in the heart and liver. It is in lower concentrations in all cells of the body, as its role is to help the mitochondria, the energy factory inside each cell, produce the power of life. (See Part I, "Coenzyme Q10.") Interestingly, CoQ10 is found in mackerel, salmon, and sardines, which also contain the highest levels of the omega-3 fatty acids touted in recent years as beneficial for a healthy cardiovascular system. It looks like a good diet for an athlete includes plenty of fish, along with the natural sources of antioxidant vitamins C and E and the antioxidant mineral selenium in whole grains, fruits, and vegetables.

There is one more reason to take antioxidants if you are a regular exerciser, particularly those of you exercising in smoggy urban areas: Ozone from heavy traffic injures lungs. According to research at the University of Massachusetts, outdoor exercise is safest in the early morning, when you can easily be seen but before the heavy traffic of rush hour.[16] And before you head for the streets, take care of your cells from the inside out. Antioxidants are your best line of internal defense against the ravages of free radicals formed by smog and by exercise.

Daily Dosage

Vitamin E	100 to 400 IU (higher dosage if exercising in mountains)
Vitamin C	1 to 3 grams
Coenzyme Q10	30 mg

Notes

1. McGuire, Rick. (1987). Lite Exercise. *Los Angeles Times*, August 25, 1.
2. Frisch, R. et al. (1985). Lower prevalence of breast cancer and cancers of the reproductive system among former college athletes compared to non-athletes. *British Journal of Cancer* 52, 885–891. Cited in Somer, Elizabeth. (1986). *The Nutrition Report*, March, 19.
3. (1983). Athletes are younger . . . and look it. *Health and Longevity Report*, August 15, 4–5.
4. Gurin, Joel, and Harris, T. George. (1987). Taking charge: The happy health-confidents. *American Health*, March, 53–57.

5. (1986). Exercise boosts body's virus-fighting proteins. *Los Angeles Times*, December 16.

6. Weyerer, S. (1992). Physical inactivity and depression in community: Evidence from the upper Bavarian field study. *International Journal of Sports Medicine* 13(6), 492–496.

7. Maranto, Gina. (1984). Exercise: How much is too much? *Discover*, October, 19–22.

8. Duthie, G., et al. (1990). Blood antioxidant status and erythrocyte lipid peroxidation following distance running. *Archives of Biochemistry* 282, 78–83.

9. Reznick, A. Z., et al. (1992). The threshold of age in exercise and antioxidants action. *Exs* 62, 423–427.

10. Cureton, Thomas Kirk. (1972) *The Physiological Effects of Wheat Germ Oil on Humans in Exercise* (p. 290). Springfield, IL: Charles C. Thomas.

11. McNaughton, Lars, and Saint-John, Mark. (1986). A review of some nutritional ergogenic aids. *International Clinical Nutrition Review*, April 6(2), 70–79.

12. Berglund, Bo. (1992). High altitude training: Aspects of hematologic adaptation. *Sports Medicine* 14(5), 289–303. Cited in Hamilton, Kirk. (1992). *Clinical Pearls* (p. 250). Sacramento, CA; ITServices. See also Simon-Schnass, Irene M. (1992). Nutrition and high altitude. *Journal of Nutrition* 122, 778–781. Cited in Hamilton, p. 254.

13. Miyashita, Mitsumasa, and Nishibata, Izumi. (1993). Nutritional supplements and athletic performance: With special reference to vitamin E. *Vitamin E—Its Usefulness in Health and in Curing Diseases* (Mino, M., et al. eds.) (pp. 153–161). Cited in Hamilton, Kirk. (1993). *Clinical Pearls* (p. 153). Sacramento, CA: ITServices.

14. Jancin, Bruce. (1993). Sports nutrition: What works and what doesn't. *Family Practice News*, September 15, 5. Cited in Hamilton (1993), p. 154.

15. Witt, E. H., et al. (1992). Exercise, oxidative damage and effects of antioxidant manipulation. *Journal of Nutrition* 122(3, Suppl.), 766–773.

16. (1983). Air pollution warning for urban joggers. *Let's Live*, January, 10.

≫ Gum Disease

Our great American high-sugar diet is certainly a factor in the gum and bone problems that together are termed periodontal disease. The beginning of tooth problems is the build-up of plaque, a combination of saliva, bacteria, and particles of food that coat the teeth and, in time, harden, particularly along the gum line. Plaque sets the stage for both tooth decay and gingivitis (an inflammation of the gums that can lead to loss of teeth). A diet high in sugar and white flour and low in essential nutrients sets the stage for plaque.

Periodontal disease is an early sign of scurvy, which is caused by vitamin C deficiency. In addition to vitamin C, it's a good idea to take bioflavonoids, which are nutrients found in nature along with vitamin C in the white rind of citrus fruit. Both strengthen capillary walls and prevent bleeding gums, fight infection, reduce inflammation, and strengthen the immune system. Vitamin A is also commonly deficient in tissues suffering periodontal disease.[1] And, surprisingly, so is the antioxidant coenzyme Q10 (CoQ10).

Imagine little engines in every cell of your body that run all cell functions. These engines have cylinders called mitochondria. Inside a mitochondrion is CoQ10, the spark that ignites the fuel to make that engine go.[2] Research suggests that taking CoQ10 supplements can also reduce periodontal inflammation and eliminate pain within the first couple weeks.[3]

According to Dr. Edward G. Wilkinson, a researcher with the

United States Air Force, with CoQ10 supplementation there was not only a reversal of gum disease, but also a regrowth of healthy tissue. The enzyme works locally and systemically to improve immune function, reduce inflammation, and protect the tissues from the toxic products of bacterial infection.[4]

Daily Dosage

Vitamin C	1,000 mg
Bioflavonoids	1,000 mg
Vitamin A	5,000 IU (or beta-carotene 5,000 IU)
Coenzyme Q10	60–75 mg, depending on the condition of the gums

Notes

1. Werbach, Melvyn R. (1993). *Nutritional Influences on Illness*, Second Edition (p. 511). Tarzana, CA: Third Line Press.
2. Bliznakov, Emile G., and Hunt, Gerald L. (1987). *The Miracle Nutrient: Coenzyme Q10* (p. 9). New York: Bantam.
3. Ibid., p.142.
4. Ibid., p. 146.

Hair Texture and Female Hair Loss

When two cysteine molecules bond together, they create a new structure, called cystine. It is in this form that cysteine contributes to the structure of proteins, such as the keratin in hair and nails. Keratin is about 12 percent cystine. When you permanent wave your hair, one solution opens these bonds to allow a second chemical solution to re-set them so your hair looks as straight or curly as you and your hairdresser desire.

If you are experiencing hair loss and no one seems to be able to diagnose why, your body may be deficient in cysteine and other sulfur-containing amino acids. Daily supplements of cysteine have increased hair shaft diameter and density of new growth in areas of the scalp experiencing human baldness and hair loss,[1] although I am sorry to say these are cases of abnormal loss, not genetically determined male pattern baldness.

You may want to ask your physician for an amino acid assay, and begin cysteine supplementation if your cystine level is low.

Other factors promoting hair loss include acute illness, poor circulation, emotional shock, iron deficiency, diabetes, thyroid disease, pharmaceuticals, radiation, and surgery.[2] The cause of the problem will dictate the cure. If poor circulation is at fault, you'll want vigorous and daily massage of the scalp, including circulation-building supplements such as vitamin E, vitamin C, Ginkgo biloba, and coenzyme Q10 (see also "Cardiovascular Disease," Part II).

Daily Dosage

Cysteine	1 to 3 grams taken twice daily (raise dose if results don't appear at the lower dose within a couple of weeks)
Vitamin C	3,000 to 10,000 mg or to bowel tolerance
Vitamin E	400 IU, increasing dosage slowly up to 1,000 IU as needed
Ginkgo biloba	180 to 300 mg

Notes

1. Braverman, Eric R., with Pfeiffer, Carl C. (1987). *The Healing Nutrients Within* (p. 91). New Canaan, CT: Keats.
2. Balch, James F., and Balch, Phyllis A. (1990). *Prescription for Nutritional Healing* (pp. 192–193). Garden City Park, NY: Avery.

Hearing Loss

Hearing is the result of the vibration of sound waves against the eardrum. Small bones behind the eardrum conduct the vibration to the cochlea in the inner ear, where these vibrations are translated into nerve impulses. The optic nerve carries the impulses to the brain. If there's a problem with the bones, there's a conductive hearing loss. If there is a problem with the nerve, there is sensorineural hearing loss. Sometimes people are bothered by a ringing noise (tinnitus) or a sensation of spinning (vertigo). Meniere's disease involves a buildup of fluid inside the ear, and can result in hearing loss, tinnitus, and vertigo.

The classic all-American high-fat high-sugar diet is perfect for reducing hearing, particularly among the aged. A high-fat diet causes a high level of fats in the blood, and these reduce the flow of oxygen and nutrients to the inner ear by making individual red blood cells both sticky and inflexible. Sugar causes the adrenal glands to release adrenalin, which constricts tiny blood vessels in the ear. According to Dr. Melvyn Werbach, "Meniere's syndrome, fluctuant hearing loss, and sudden deafness have all been shown to be associated with abnormal responses to sugar. In these disorders, replacement of sugar and other refined carbohydrates with either a high-protein or an unrefined, complex-carbohydrate diet is sometimes followed by a lessening of symptoms."[1]

Vitamin A, on which the cochlea is dependent, is particularly important for healthy hearing. In one experiment, 300 people with hearing loss were injected with vitamin A, and 83 percent reported improved hearing. Vitamin E helps vitamin A do its job. Says Werbach of vitamins A and E, "Particularly when the auditory symptoms are related to aging, the combination may cause a measurable improvement in hearing."[2] A third nutrient that can improve hearing is Ginkgo biloba, which increases blood circulation. Ginkgo is quite safe and has helped tinnitus, vertigo, and acute cochlear deafness in double-blind research studies.

Daily Dosage

Vitamin A	20,000 IU
Vitamin E	400 IU
Ginkgo biloba	120 mg (divided into two or three doses)

Notes

1. Werbach, Melvyn. (1993). *Healing Through Nutrition* (p. 218). New York: Harper Collins.
2. Ibid., p. 219.

Heavy Metal Toxicity

Cysteine is an amino acid, a building block of protein, which can reduce copper, cobalt, and lead toxicity. Cysteine combines with copper and can reverse copper overdose in the blood and pull the copper out of certain organs. According to Drs. Braverman and Pfeiffer, "Copper toxicity is an ever-present danger in the United States." They blame copper in water pipes, poultry, and pig feed (as an antifungal agent and growth enhancer). They also note that although some copper is essential for health, excess copper can cause psychosis and other mental disturbances.[1]

Lead contributes to lowered intelligence in children and hypertension in adults. Lead is in the environment as residues of leaded gasoline. It is still found in the soil near roadways and is tracked into homes on shoes. In addition, lead contaminates people indoors by leaching into their food from leaded ceramic glazes on pottery and is absorbed through the skin or licked off fingers by babies and young children playing on the floor around windowsills and walls with old, chipped paint. It is swallowed by young and old in drinking water. In 1986, the Environmental Protection Agency surveyed lead exposure and concluded up to 40 percent of the lead threatening Americans is brought to them in their drinking water, through lead solder, particularly in copper pipes.[2] Turn-of-the-century plumbing may be made entirely of lead! Lead poisoning in America's inner cities is serious and wide-

170

spread. In addition to cysteine, lead can be drawn out of the body with selenium, high doses of vitamin C,[3] and a high fiber diet.

Daily Dosage

Cysteine	1 to 3 grams
Selenium	200 mcg
Vitamin C	3 to 10 grams or to bowel tolerance

Notes

1. Braverman, Eric R., and Pfeiffer, Carl C. (1987). *The Healing Nutrients Within* (p. 115). New Canaan, CT: Keats.
2. Reuben, Carolyn. (1992). *The Healthy Baby Book: A Parent's Guide to Preventing Birth Defects and Other Long-Term Medical Problems Before, During, and After Pregnancy* (p. 87). Los Angeles: Jeremy P. Tarcher/Perigee.
3. Rimland, Bernard, and Larson, Gerald E. (1981). The manpower quality decline: An ecological perspective. *Armed Forces and Society* 8(1), 62.

✎ HIV Infection/AIDS

Acquired Immune Deficiency Syndrome (AIDS) is thought to be a virally induced affront to the immune system that allows otherwise mild conditions to overwhelm the health of the person infected. The virus generally thought to be the main cause of AIDS is called the Human Immunodeficiency Virus (HIV). Although there is no known "cure" for AIDS, in a few infected individuals both the virus and antibodies previously found in the blood disappear, indicating the person has rid his or her body of the infection before AIDS developed.[1]

Some research links reactive oxygen species, meaning molecules that cause oxidation, to the progression of HIV infection, as well as to the side effects caused by azidothymidine (AZT), the one drug currently approved for treatment of AIDS. For example, when researchers checked for intracellular glutathione in the white blood cells of HIV-positive patients, they found a lower measure of this antioxidant than in healthy controls. Glutathione is used by glutathione peroxidase, the major antioxidant enzyme that removes hydrogen peroxide from the body. Hydrogen peroxide removal is particularly important to patients with AIDS, as the toxin can inhibit T-lymphocyte activity and can damage lymphocytes in a significant way. Glutathione deficiency is thought to play an important role in the progression of the disease.[2]

Vitamin C and HIV Infection

In the January 27, 1990, issue of *The Lancet*, Dr. Robert Cathcart III published his experience treating over 250 HIV-positive patients with very high doses of vitamin C. Cathcart found his sickest patients could tolerate between 100 to 200 grams per day in hourly divided dosages. According to Cathcart, the correct dose of vitamin C for any condition is that dose which is just under the dose that causes loose stool. He finds the correct dose by increasing the grams consumed until loose stools result, then cuts back on the dosage until the problem ends. He has coined the term "bowel tolerance dose" to identify this phenomenon.

Cathcart used intravenous sodium ascorbate with the HIV-positive patients, dripped over 3 to 4 hours, one to three times daily, along with oral vitamin C. Cathcart maintains that such enormous doses of vitamin C help create the body's premier antioxidant enzyme, glutathione peroxidase, and the result in his patients is a maintenance of CD4 T-cells (immune cells that are depleted in HIV infection), reduced lymph swelling, more energy, and reduced allergic reactions to antibiotics.[3]

During his 24 years of experience using such massive doses of vitamin C for some 22,000 patients with complaints ranging from severe colds to AIDS, Cathcart has found that patients such as those with AIDS who suffer chronic diarrhea actually improve bowel function with appropriately high doses of vitamin C, until the "bowel tolerance" dose is reached.

Other clinicians have also reported positive results using such massive doses of vitamin C, including the elimination of Kaposi's sarcoma.[4]

Other Antioxidants and HIV

Frank Stall and colleagues encourage the use of *N*-acetylcysteine (NAC, a pharmaceutical form of the amino acid cysteine) to fight the HIV retrovirus, as NAC is a nontoxic therapy that will help replace missing glutathione.[5] NAC works synergistically with vitamin C, meaning there is greater benefit in taking the two supplements together than either one alone.

In other reports, 27 percent of HIV-positive patients with lymph gland involvement were found deficient in vitamin E; cells infected with HIV were found low in superoxide dismutase, an especially powerful antioxidant enzyme; and people with AIDS have been found low in selenium in heart and blood. In one study, 400 mcg of selenium per day was given to 20 AIDS patients in the form of selenium yeast. Their blood levels of selenium returned to normal in 70 days, and 14 of the patients reported improved gastrointestinal function, improved appetite, improved memory and concentration, improved libido, and improved mood as well as enhanced natural killer cell activity. Only two of the twenty patients reported feeling worse, and four felt no change.[6]

Dr. Richard D. Semba and colleagues studied vitamin A levels in 179 HIV-infected subjects. Compared to controls, those infected with HIV had lower vitamin A levels, lower CD4 helper cells, and higher mortality The authors conclude that vitamin A status seems to be an important risk factor for disease progression in cases of HIV infection.[7]

When Alice M. Tang and colleagues at The Johns Hopkins University followed asymptomatic HIV-positive men for 7 years, they found those consuming from about 9,000 to about 20,000 IU of vitamin A and more than 715 mg of vitamin C a day were about 50 percent less likely to develop fullblown AIDS than those who consumed lower doses of these nutrients. (The healthier men also consumed more than 61 mg of niacin, but not more than 20 mg of zinc, daily.) These researchers noted a U-shaped curve of vitamin A intake, with those taking the lowest and highest doses more likely to develop AIDS. According to the researchers, the benefit of these particular nutrients may be due to their antioxidant and immune-system-stimulating effects.[8]

Tang's wasn't the only study to show a benefit of improving antioxidant levels in people who are HIV positive or who have AIDS. Beta-carotene supplementation was used in one double-blind, placebo-controlled trial with 21 HIV-positive patients. Participants were given 180 mg of beta-carotene or a placebo per day for 4 weeks, then the supplements were switched for the next 4 weeks. There was a statistically significant rise in white blood cell count and a percent change in CD4 helper cells and in the CD4–CD8 ratio among those taking the beta-carotene compared to placebo. The absolute level of helper cells and the CD4–CD8 ratio did rise with beta-carotene supplementation, but was not statistically significant. The investigators concluded that beta-carotene appears to have an immunostimulating effect among HIV-positive patients.[9]

Recently, the herb Ginkgo biloba has been found useful in laboratory experiments against *pneumocystis carinii*, an opportunistic lung infection common in AIDS.[10]

Not everyone is enthusiastic about people with AIDS taking megadoses of antioxidants. Drs. Barry Halliwell and Carroll E. Cross of the University of California, Davis, suggest that low levels of free radicals have certain benefits to the immune system in regard to lymphocyte function, and there may be harmful effects of overly enthusiastic consumption of antioxidants.[11] They recommend emphasizing dietary intake of amino acids, vitamins, and minerals and minimizing supplementation.

Daily Dosage

Vitamin A	10,000 IU
Vitamin C	to bowel tolerance
Bioflavonoids	1,000 mg
Vitamin E	400 IU
Selenium	50 to 200 mcg
NAC or L-cysteine	400 mg
Ginkgo biloba	180 mg

Notes

1. Clayman, Charles B. (ed.) (1989). *The American Medical Association Encyclopedia of Medicine* (p. 76). New York: Random House.

2. Stall, Frank, et al. (1992). Glutathione deficiency and human immunodeficiency virus infection. *The Lancet* 339, 909–912.

3. Cathcart, Robert F., III. (1990). Glutathione and HIV infection. *The Lancet* 335, 235.
4. Cathcart, Robert F., III. (1990). Glutathione and HIV infection. *The Lancet* 335, 235. Brighthope, I. (1987). AIDS-remissions using nutrient therapies and megadose intravenous ascorbate. *International Clinical Nutrition Reviews* 7(2), 53–75.
5. Stall, pp. 909–912.
6. Shamberger, Raymond J. (1992). Selenium and the antioxidant defense system. *Journal of Advancement in Medicine* 5(1), 7–19.
7. Semba, Richard D., et al. (1993). Increased mortality associated with vitamin A deficiency during human immunodeficiency virus type 1 infection. *Archives of Internal Medicine* 153, 2149–2154.
8. Tang, Alice M., et al. (1993). Dietary micronutrient intake and risk of progression to acquired immunodeficiency syndrome (AIDS) in human immunodeficiency virus type 1 (HIV-1)-infected homosexual men. *American Journal of Epidemiology* 138(11), 937–951.
9. Coodley, Gregg O., et al. (1993). "Beta-carotene in HIV infection. *Journal of Acquired Immune Deficiency Syndromes* 6, 272–276.
10. Murray, Michael T. (1990). Ginkgo biloba: The living fossil, Part 2. *Phyto-Pharmica Review* 3(4), 1.
11. Halliwell, Barry, and Cross, Carroll E. (1991). Reactive oxygen species, antioxidants, and acquired immunodeficiency syndrome: Sense or speculation? *Archives of Internal Medicine* 151(1), 29–31.

⚞⚟ Immune Dysfunction

When we think of blood we usually think of the color red, but our bloodstream hosts legions of white blood cells that defend us from bacteria, viruses, and foreign proteins of various kinds. These blood cells are the core of our immune system, and the quality of our health is directly related to their vitality.

How well the immune system functions can be measured in a variety of ways. For example, Johns Hopkins School of Hygiene and Public Health supervised a study of 236 Indonesian preschool-age children given vitamin A before taking the diphtheria–pertussis–tetanus vaccine. Some children had a slight vitamin A deficiency before receiving the injection. Others had what was considered adequate vitamin A. Both groups showed significant improvement in their immune system function, as measured by blood tests, compared to those children given a placebo.[1]

Vitamin A clearly enhances the body's immune system by increasing the response of T and B lymphocytes to biological invaders of various sorts. Writing in the *Bulletin of the World Health Organization* in 1992, J. H. Humphrey estimates that 124 million children worldwide are vitamin A deficient, and improvement in their vitamin A status could prevent as many as 500,000 deaths among infants and 2 million deaths among children ages 1 to 4, as well as reduce the incidence of diarrhea, respiratory disease, infections, and measles.[2]

Vitamin E is another useful therapy for improving immune system functioning. According to Dr. Jeffrey B. Blumberg, director of the Antioxidant Research Laboratory, USDA Human Nutrition Research Center on Aging at Tufts University, high levels of vitamin E in the bloodstream parallel fewer infections in adults over the age of 60.

Dosages of 300 mg to 1,600 IU of vitamin E per day have been beneficial in various experiments, enhancing production of antibodies and, at least in animal experiments, enhancing resistance to bacterial and viral infections.[3] Among humans, the elderly are particularly susceptible to lipid peroxidation (oxidation of fatty acids in the bloodstream and elsewhere)[4] and need to strengthen their immune function, to prevent chronic disease.[5]

If you have recurring infections, you probably need more vitamin E than you are currently consuming. (When 100 healthy people over age 60 were interviewed regarding their nutritional intake and rate of infection, there was a statistically significant parallel between the level of vitamin E in their blood and the number of infections they suffered during the past 3 years.)[6] Vitamin E isn't only for adults. In a study of Canadian children around age 3, low levels of vitamin E were associated with laboratory-based lower levels of immunity.[7] Whatever the age, it seems that high levels of vitamin E in the bloodstream help keep us free of infections. However, the exact mechanism by which the vitamin accomplishes this feat is still unknown.

When selenium is deficient, immunity is impaired, particularly when vitamin E is also deficient.

In addition, vitamin C in doses of from 1 to 3 grams per day also improves immune response.[8]

Daily Dosage

Vitamin C	1 to 3 grams or to bowel tolerance
Vitamin E	100 to 400 IU (confer with a nutritionally trained medical provider for higher doses)
Selenium	50 to 200 mcg depending on severity of condition

Notes

1. Semba, R. et al. (1992). Depressed immune response to tetanus in children with vitamin A deficiency. *Journal of Nutrition* 122, 101–107.
2. Humphrey, J.H., et al. (1992). Vitamin A deficiency and attributable mortality among under-five-year-olds. *Bulletin of the World Health Organization* 70(2), 225–232.
3. Blumberg, Jeffrey B. (1993). The role of vitamin E in immunity during aging. In *Vitamin E—Its Usefulness in Health and Diseases* (Mino, M., et al., eds.) (pp. 219–229). Farmington, CT: S. Karger.
4. Meydani, M. (1992). Vitamin E requirement in relation to dietary fish oil and oxidative stress in elderly. *Exs* 62, 411–418.
5. Meydani, S. N. (1993). Vitamin/mineral supplementation, the aging immune response, and risk of infection. *Nutrition Reviews* 51(4), 106–109.
6. Chavance, M., et al. (1984). Immunologic and nutritional status among the elderly. In *Lymphoid Cell Function in Aging* (deWeck, A.L., ed.). Rijswijk, The Netherlands: Evrage (1993). In *Nutritional Influences on Illness, Second Edition* (Werbach, M. R., ed.) (p.359). Tarzana, CA: Third Line Press.
7. Bendich, Adrianne. (1993). Vitamin E and human immune functions. *Human Nutrition—A Comprehensive Treatise* 8 (Chapter 10), 217–228. In Hamilton, Kirk (ed.). (1993). *Clinical Pearls* (p. 183). Sacramento, CA: ITServices.
8. Anderson, R. (1984). The immunostimulatory, anti-inflammatory and anti-allergic properties of ascorbate. *Advances in Nutrition Research* 6, 19–45. Cited in Werbach, Melvyn R. (1991). *Nutritional Influences on Illness, Second Edition* (p. 357). Tarzana, CA: Third Line Press.

~~~ Infertility

Veterinarians and breeders have been among the pioneers in using nutrients to improve fertility. For example, the relationship of beta-carotene and fertility has been closely researched in animals. The fact that the nutrient is found in large measure in ovaries and adrenal glands lead researchers to believe there must be some connection between reproduction and beta-carotene. With dairy cattle, the nutrient seems to stimulate greater progesterone production. If this carries over into human physiology, it might be of great interest to those women struggling with infertility due to low progesterone. Certainly, in cows, increased fertility follows supplementing the animal's diet with beta-carotene.[1]

Vitamin A also promotes fertility by contributing to the production of sperm. And hypogonadism (underdevelopment of sex organs) is a clinical sign of vitamin A deficiency.

Research is slight but of enough significance to note that in mice[2] and in men[3] studies show a relationship between levels of selenium and healthy sperm. With the mice, there was significant abnormality in the selenium-deficient sperm. In men, sperm count was significantly lower in cases in which the level of selenium in the blood serum was low.

Healthy sperm are a product of a healthy internal and external environment. If you are exposed to toxic substances such as chemicals or radiation (even the nonionizing kind) at the workplace or while pursuing your hobbies, take the steps necessary to protect yourself.

Nutritionally, the antioxidants that help the liver detoxify your body from pollutants (including recreational drugs) are needed in liberal measure if you have a low sperm count. For example, 75 smokers in their 20s and 30s who smoke at least one pack a day were given a 200- or 1,000-mg dose of vitamin C or a placebo. The most significant improvement in sperm quality occurred in those taking 1,000 mg of the vitamin, but even the 200-mg dose helped more than the placebo.[4]

Daily Dosage

Vitamin A	10,000 IU
Beta-carotene	5,000 IU
Vitamin C	1 to 3 grams or to bowel tolerance
Vitamin E	400 IU
Selenium	50 mcg

Notes

1. Folman, Y., et al. (1983). The effect of dietary and climatic factors on fertility and on plasma progesterone and oestradiol-17 beta levels in dairy cows. *Journal of Steroid Biochemistry* 19, 863–868.
2. Watanabe, T., and Endo, A. (1991). Effects of selenium deficiency on sperm morphology and spermatocyte chromosomes in mice. *Mutation Research* 262(2), 93–99.
3. Kranjavi, H., et al. (1992). Selenium and fertility in men. *Trace Elements in Medicine* 9(2), 107–108. Cited in Hamilton, Kirk. (1992). *Clinical Pearls* (p. 258). Sacramento, CA: ITServices.
4. Dawson, Earl B., et al. (1992). Effect of ascorbic acid supplementation on the sperm quality of smokers. *Fertility and Sterility* 58(5), 1034–1039. Cited in Hamilton, Kirk. (1993). *Clinical Pearls* (p. 159). Sacramento, CA: ITServices.

Intermittent Claudication

Claudication means limping. *Intermittent claudication* refers to a pain in the calf so severe it interferes with walking, but disappears with rest. It is caused by inadequate blood supply, which may be due to blockage by plaque or a clot, by spasms of the muscles around a blood vessel, or by a hardened vessel that can't move the blood appropriately. Regular exercise is extremely effective therapy for intermittent claudication, improving walking ability in over 80 percent of patients.

Two good antioxidant herbal therapies for the problem are garlic and Ginkgo biloba. A group of 32 people with intermittent claudication were given 800 mg daily of garlic powder and compared to a control group the same size. After the fifth week of treatment, there was a drop in diastolic blood pressure, a decrease in blood viscosity and tendency to clot, and a drop in cholesterol among the garlic takers. They also could walk significantly farther than the placebo group.[1]

Ginkgo biloba leaves decrease blood viscosity and tendency to clot and increase blood flow in capillaries. Of 15 controlled trials using ginkgo for intermittent claudication, all showed positive results and no serious side effects were reported. In most trials, 120 to 160 mg a day was used, divided into three doses. One of the two best trials found subjects improving walking distance by 110 meters after 6 months of ginkgo therapy, compared to only 31 meters for those consuming a placebo during that time.[2] Treatment did not show its greatest benefit until 4 to 6 weeks after treatment began. It is unknown at this time whether a higher dose would be useful or whether the benefits remain after treatment ceases.

The one antioxidant vitamin studied for intermittent claudication is vitamin E, which seems to be our wonder treatment for any cardiovascular complaint. One representative study was published by Haeger in 1973; patients using vitamin E increased walking distance 54 percent compared with 23 percent for controls.[3]

What happens if you consume garlic, ginkgo, *and* vitamin E? Try it, and be sure to let your cardiologist know! He/she may want to write you up in the medical literature.

Daily Dosage

Vitamin E	100 to 400 IU
Garlic	800 mg (you may want to use a deodorized brand)
Ginkgo biloba	120–180 mg

Notes

1. Kiesewetter, H., et al. (1993). Effects of garlic coated tablets in peripheral arterial occlusive disease. *Clinical Investigator* 71, 383–386. Cited in Hamilton, Kirk. (1993). *Clinical Pearls* (p.192). Sacramento, CA: ITServices.
2. Kleijnen, Jos, and Knipschild, Paul. (1992). Ginkgo biloba. *The Lancet* 340, 1136–1139.
3. Haeger, K. (1973). Walking distance and arterial flow during longterm treatment of intermittent claudication with alpha-tocopherol. *Vasa* 2, 280–287.

Measles

Measles is one of the most severe infectious diseases among the poor children of the world. In fact, the disease kills about 2 million children a year, particularly in developing countries. In these countries measles mortality is associated with secondary complications such as pneumonia, other respiratory diseases, diarrhea, malnutrition, and blindness.[1]

In a study in South Africa, 189 children admitted to the Red Cross War Memorial Children's Hospital in Rondebosch received either 400,000 units of vitamin A or a placebo after the measles rash appeared. Those on vitamin A recovered more rapidly from pneumonia and diarrhea, and were less hoarse. Ten of the 12 children who died were not taking vitamin A. The risk of death or major complication during the hospital stay of the children supplemented with vitamin A was half that of the control group.

In one randomized, double-blind, placebo-controlled study, 60 African children ages 2 to 4 years old were hospitalized with measles complicated by pneumonia and diarrhea. Subjects received either a large dose of vitamin A as recommended by the World Health Organization (WHO) or a placebo. As a result, diarrhea was reduced by 82 percent, herpes by 61 percent, and respiratory tract infection decreased by 85 percent in the supplemented group. In addition, weight gain by the sixth week was significant in the supplemented group as compared to the placebo group.

Measles depletes already low vitamin A reserves. In addition, vitamin A deficiency contributes to morbidity and mortality in children. In an Indonesian study, even mild signs of vitamin A deficiency in preschool-age children were associated with a four-fold increase in mortality; the incidence of diarrhea and respiratory disease was increased two- to threefold.[2] The authors of this study recommend that all children be given vitamin A if they have severe measles, regardless of whether they are deficient in the vitamin. According to one report author, Dr. A. Sommer, from Johns Hopkins University, "It is now estimated that improving the vitamin A status of all deficient children worldwide would prevent 1–3 million childhood deaths annually."

A joint WHO/UNICEF statement urges "High dosage vitamin A supplementation should be provided to all children diagnosed with measles in communities in which vitamin A deficiency is a recognized problem." The research seems to indicate that the level of vitamin A at the time the measles develops is what is most important.

Although vitamin A is too toxic for parents to give to their children without a physician's supervision, public health officials might use vitamin A with good results in areas where poverty is rampant and measles are most dangerous. What parents can safely do on their own is make sure their children eat at least five fresh fruits and vegetables every day to maintain a healthy level of vitamin A (because adequate vitamin A will be created from the beta-carotene in those fruits and vegetables).

Daily Dosage

Vitamin A   Five fresh fruits and vegetables per day, for adequate beta-carotene, a plant source of vitamin A. Consult with your medical provider for recommendations on supplementation.

Notes

1. *The Lancet* (editorial) (1987). Vitamin A for measles. *The Lancet* 1(8541), 1067–1068.
2. Sommer, Alfred, et al. (1983). Increased mortality in children with mild vitamin A deficiency. *The Lancet* 2 (8350), 585–588.

Memory Loss/Senility

Two changes in the brain conspire to reduce memory: a change in the ability of nerves to transmit quality information down the nerve fiber and across the synapse (space) between nerves, and a change in blood flow quantity, quality, or both. Nerves and blood are what form the bottom line of memory.

To help improve nerve transmission, you can use the antioxidant amino acids L-cysteine and L-methionine. To help improve blood vessel health and blood quantity and quality, you can use vitamin E, bioflavonoids, and ginkgo biloba (see Part I, "Ginkgo Biloba").

Memory loss can occur at any age, but senility is, by definition, related to old age. Dr. Abram Hoffer, with the help of medical journalist Morton Walker, has written an entire book on the subject, titled *Nutrients to Age Without Senility*.[1] They make a strong case for lifestyle factors, particularly nutritional deficiencies, as the root of many cases of senility, rather than advancing age. They point out that Michelangelo sculpted the Pieta when he was eighty and Disraeli became one of Britain's most notable prime ministers when he was seventy. There are plenty of examples of people whose minds were sharp and effective into their nineties. Hoffer and Walker hypothesize that senility is caused by lack of enough oxygen and nourishment in brain cells. They believe that if given adequate oxygen and nourishment, no one will become senile.

One form of senility is especially feared: Alzheimer's disease, a progressive deterioration of nerve cells. It involves years of increasingly failing mental capabilities and is only conclusively diagnosed by autopsy.

Alzheimer's disease was a rare condition in 1907, when it was first described. Today, it is the most common cause of dementia, perhaps a sad commentary on the unhealthy lifestyle and polluted world that has been created over the past 90 years. There is one ray of light, however. It appears ginkgo biloba prevents continued deterioration of mental capacities, even in Alzheimer's disease, and is most useful in the early stages of the disease.[2] For example, in a double-blind study of elderly patients who did not have Alzheimer's, ginkgo improved performance on tests of mental acuity and memory, and those patients with the most deteriorated initial condition improved the most.[3]

Two Dutch researchers reviewed 40 controlled trials of ginkgo for cerebral insufficiency and found eight of good quality.[4] In all studies, those taking the ginkgo enjoyed results clearly superior to those obtained by the controls and reported only mild, if any, side effects.

According to Hoffer and Walker,[5] in order to prevent senility and the mental confusion that is its foundation, you must reduce the formation of free radicals by avoiding radiation, cigarette smoke, and toxic elements; increase consumption of fruits and vegetables that contain liberal doses of free radical scavengers such as The Four ACES; and take specific nutritional supplements. Please see the recommendations that follow.

Daily Dosage

Vitamin C	take to bowel tolerance
Vitamin E	800 IU[6]
L-Cysteine	500 mg twice a day
L-Methionine	1 gram
Ginkgo biloba	100 to 800 mg (start at the lower dose for several weeks, and increase only if needed).

Notes

1. Hoffer, Abram, and Walker, Morton. (1980) *Nutrients to Age Without Senility* (pp. 129–152). New Canaan, CT: Keats.

2. Funfgeld, E. W. (1989). A natural and broad spectrum neotropic substance for treatment of SDAT—The ginkgo biloba extract. In Murray, Frank. (1993). *Ginkgo Biloba* (p. 20). New Canaan, CT: Keats.

3. Murray, Michael T. (1990). Ginkgo Biloba: The living fossil, part 2. *Phyto-Pharmica Review* 3(4), 1.

4. Kleijnen, Jos, and Knipschild, Paul. (1992). Ginkgo biloba. *The Lancet* 340, 1136–1139.

5. Hoffer and Walker (1980), p. 134.

6. Hoffer claims he has seen Huntington's chorea reversed using 800 IU of vitamin E per day, even though Huntington's chorea is considered to be a genetically inherited degenerative muscle-wasting disease with no known cure. Hoffer and Walker, p. 149.

⟋ Night Blindness/Reduced Daylight Vision

One of the most ancient medical texts in the world, the Eber's Papyrus (written in 1500 B.C.), advises eating roasted ox liver to cure night blindness. Over a thousand years later, on the Greek island of Cos, Hippocrates recommended consuming the ox liver raw for the same purpose (we don't have a record of how many patients opted for night blindness). In central Africa, medical authorities suggested eating chicken livers to improve night vision. It took until the twentieth century for scientists to discover vitamin A and then connect the fact that the liver, as the storehouse of vitamin A, is therefore useful in curing night blindness.

At the back of our eyeball is a special area called the retina. Inside the retina are rod-shaped cells that contain a light-sensitive protein called rhodopsin, or visual purple. Visual purple is essential to night vision. An essential component of visual purple is vitamin A. Night blindness is a symptom of mild vitamin A deficiency.

Could squeezing liver juice onto the eye cure night blindness? Contemporary doctors say this might be possible, if applied frequently enough, because the liver extract contains enough vitamin A to pass through the tear ducts into the digestive system. Cod liver oil (taken orally) can also cure night blindness, since it is a rich source of vitamin A.[1]

The more visual purple in the rod cells, the sharper your vision at night. Visual purple is used up too quickly to be regenerated in daylight, but in dim light rhodopsin can be regenerated. Bilberry, a member of the blueberry family, quickens the body's ability to regenerate visual purple and improves night vision (see Part I, "Bilberry").

The first simple study of bilberry and visual purple took place in 1964 and involved 37 subjects. They took bilberry extract before their visual acuity and adaptation to dim light were measured. The greatest measures of improvement occurred 4 hours after consuming bilberry, and disappeared about 24 hours later.

Some people are less able to see in bright sunlight than in dimmer light. One intrepid researcher measured the response of people with this problem (called hemeralopia, or day blindness) to bilberry supplementation and found that subjects experienced less sensitivity to light by the second day of the experiment. After the course of treatment, the reduced sensitivity gradually declined back to their normal hypersensitive condition, suggesting that continued use of bilberry is necessary to maintain its benefits.

During daylight, bilberry seems to work on the eye in a different way than does regenerating visual purple. The herb appears able to magnify or enhance the perception of light reaching the retina, so a clearer image results.

Daily Dosage

Cod liver oil	1 tablespoon
Bilberry	60 to 180 mg to prevent night or day blindness; increase dosage slowly up to 300 mg for chronic conditions.

Note

1. Maumenee, Edward A. (1993). The history of vitamin A and its ophthalmic implications: A personal viewpoint. *Archives of Ophthalmology* 111, 547–550.

Osteoarthritis

Arthron is Greek for joint; *–itis* means inflammation. Arthritis is a general term for inflammed joints. The condition is often painful, and sometimes disfiguring. Osteoarthritis is a localized degeneration of one or more joints, which may be painful without being inflammed. Rheumatoid arthritis, in contrast, is also painful but is by definition an inflammatory disease that often results in deformation of bone and atrophy of muscle.

In general, a diet perfect for exacerbating arthritis is the usual American fare: lots of meat, sugar, refined carbohydrates, salt, and coffee. In contrast, the diet that helps reverse arthritis includes low-fat meals of mostly vegetables and fresh vegetable juices, cold-water fish (rich in omega-3 fatty acids) and New Zealand green-lipped mussels, and whole grains (a good source of both vitamin E and the B complex).

It is critical in cases of arthritis of any kind to investigate the possibility of food sensitivities. Some people with osteoarthritis, for example, are especially sensitive to vegetables in the nightshade family (tomatoes, potatoes, eggplant, and peppers) and find noticeable relief when they eliminate these foods. If the sensitivities cannot be eliminated by conventional desensitization procedures in an allergist's office, by acupuncture and herbs in the office of a state-licensed acupuncturist, or by the use of nontoxic homeopathic remedies,[1] the offending foods should be eliminated from the diet permanently.

Vitamin A can be deficient in connective tissue diseases, and the nutrient is essential for the proper development and maintenance of cartilage. The same is true of vitamin C.

Vitamin E was used in a single-blind study (where the physician knows who receives the vitamin and who the placebo but the patients don't know). Twenty-nine patients with osteoarthritis took part, with 52 percent of those taking vitamin E feeling less pain, compared to 4 percent of those taking a placebo.[2] Vitamin E has been found effective in at least two double-blind studies (where neither the doctors nor the patients know which group is taking the vitamin or the placebo). Alpha tocopherol seems to inhibit production of substances called prostaglandins that cause inflammation.

Methionine is an antioxidant amino acid, which in one double-blind experiment proved more effective than ibuprofen (Motrin) as a pain reliever for patients with osteoarthritis.[3]

Daily Dosage

Vitamin A	10,000 IU
Vitamin C	starting at 1 gram, increase dosage to bowel tolerance
Vitamin E	600 IU
Methionine	250 mg four times a day

Notes

1. For information about homeopathic remedies, read *Everybody's Guide to Homeopathic Medicines*, by Stephen Cummings and Dana Ullman (1991), New York: Putnam, or contact Homeopathic Educational Services, 2036 Blake Street, Berkeley, CA 94704 (510-649-0294).

2. Machtey, I., and Ouaknine, L. (1978). Tocopherol in osteoarthritis: A controlled pilot study. *Journal of the American Geriatric Society* 26, 328. Cited in Werbach, Melvyn R. (1993). *Nutritional Influences on Illness, Second Edition* (p. 466). Tarzana, CA: Third Line Press.

3. Marcolongo, R., et al. (1985). Double-blind multicentre study of the activity of S-adenosyl-methionine in hip osteoarthritis. *Current Therapeutic Research* 37, 82–94. Cited in Murray, Michael, and Pizzorno, Joseph. (1991). Rheumatoid arthritis. In *Encyclopedia of Natural Medicine* (p. 450). Rocklin, CA: Prima Publishing.

〰️ Rheumatoid Arthritis

Rheumatoid arthritis (RA) is a systemic autoimmune disease. The body reacts against its own cells, causing an inflammation and thickening of joints that often results in the deformation of bone and the atrophy of muscle, accompanied by a great deal of chronic pain. A rheumatoid factor is sometimes measurable in the blood, which, when found, confirms the diagnosis.

The exact cause of RA is unknown. Altered permeability of the intestines might be part of the answer because this could lead to the absorption of substances the body perceives as invaders that are similar in structure to substances in joint tissues. The body thinks it must attack the invaders, and it attacks its own joints in the process.[1]

One way the joints are damaged is by free radical attacks. Thus, a number of studies attempt to stop pain and halt the progress of the disease by using free radical scavengers in strong doses.

In Israel, doctors were surprised when they read in a study of fish oil for rheumatoid arthritis that some members of a control group given a "placebo" that contained just 3 mg of vitamin E in coconut oil felt improvement in their pain. So, the doctors tried giving a higher dose of vitamin E (600 mg per day) to patients with rheumatoid arthritis. Fifteen of the 29 people taking vitamin E reported significant improvement, compared to only one of those taking a different placebo.[2] When 1,200 mg per day of d-alpha-tocopherol acetate was given to people with RA or osteoarthritis of the knee and hip, only those with rheumatoid arthritis reported receiving pain relief. It appears that vitamin E has an anti-inflammatory effect on RA.[3]

It is known that vitamin E works synergistically with selenium, as well as with antioxidant enzymes such as catalase, glutathione peroxidase, and superoxide dismutase. Patients with RA and chronic juvenile arthritis tend to have low selenium levels in their blood. In fact, the lower the selenium level, the more severe the disease. In one study published in 1984, a combination of vitamin E and selenium was successful in reducing symptoms of RA.[4] The same journal published another study on selenium and arthritis in 1985. This study found selenium levels significantly lower in patients with RA than in controls.[5]

Vitamin C is useful for RA because it can reduce inflammation and increase the activity of superoxide dismutase, a free radical scavenging enzyme.

Bioflavonoids are another antioxidant useful for fighting RA. Some bioflavonoids reduce inflammation by lowering production of leukotrienes. According to Drs. Michael Murray and Joseph Pizzorno, bioflavonoids are best taken between meals with pancreatic enzymes or bromelain (both are digestive aids) and vitamin C. This combination, they say, has resulted in better pain relief than even nonsteroidal drugs such as aspirin and indomethacin.[6]

Daily Dosage

Vitamin E	400 IU
Vitamin C	1 to 3 grams, taken in small doses throughout the day
Selenium	200 mcg
Bioflavonoids	1 gram
Pancreatin	350 mg at least a half hour after each meal
Bromelain	250 mg at least a half hour after each meal

Notes

1. Murray, Michael, and Pizzorno, Joseph. (1991). Rheumatoid arthritis. In *Encyclopedia of Natural Medicine* (p. 493). Rocklin, CA: Prima Publishing.

2. Machtey, I. (1991). Vitamin E and arthritis/Vitamin E and rheumatoid arthritis. *Arthritis and Rheumatism* 34(9), 1205. Cited in Hamilton, Kirk. (1992).Clinical Pearls (p. 56). Sacramento, CA: ITServices.

3. *Ibid.*

4. Munthe, E., and Aseth, J. (1984). Treatment of rheumatoid arthritis with selenium and vitamin E. *Scandinavian Journal of Rheumatology* 1984, 53 (Suppl.), 103. Cited in Murray and Pizzorno, p. 495.

5. Tarp, U., et al. (1985). Low selenium level in severe rheumatoid arthritis. *Scandinavian Journal of Rheumatology* 14, 97–101. Cited in Garrison, Robert, Jr. (ed.). (1986). *The Nutrition Report*, January, 2.

6. Murray and Pizzorno, p. 496.

Sexual Dysfunction

Older men, in general, need longer intervals between acts of intercourse than do younger men, but intercourse isn't all there is to sex! In fact, women often complain about a lack of foreplay during lovemaking, thus older men, using time to their favor, can be the most satisfying of lovers.

"Your body," writes Dr. Cynthia Mervis Watson in *Love Potions*, "is designed to thrive on movement. Like a machine that has been left idle for months, the sedentary body becomes 'rusty' and difficult to crank up."[1] In her excellent book, Watson describes many studies on middle aged men and women linking regular aerobic activity with greater sex drive and more frequent orgasms. Exercise also is a successful cure for fatigue, anxiety, and depression, which can dampen libido at any age.

A slow filling of the penis with blood may be due to congestion of small blood vessels in the penis. A high fat, high sugar diet is not conducive to clean blood vessels. A cause of lack of interest in sex is fatigue. Frequent use of caffeine, sugar, and refined carbohydrates such as white flour can lead to fatigue and to headache, depression, and moodiness—all common reasons why people resist having sex, even when they have a willing partner. Vitamin C is one antioxidant associated with improvement of fatigue.[2]

Vitamins C and E will help improve circulation. Also consider ginkgo biloba, which studies have proven increases blood circulation in the legs and head, so one expects it must increase blood circulation midway in between as well. Happily, studies prove this to be true.[3]

Homeopathic remedies are natural substances that have been diluted many times with water and shaken vigorously in a laboratory technique called succussion. These remedies are available over the counter at health food stores, food cooperatives, specialized pharmacies, and some large drugstore chains. According to Dr. Watson, homeopathic selenium "can be efficacious to the sexual organs, especially in men when there is increased sexual desire with loss of erections." Some symptoms Watson says respond well to homeopathic selenium include feelings of fatigue and melancholy, memory loss, and insomnia. "Men with prostatic enlargement or who are prone to premature ejaculation may benefit from homeopathic doses of selenium."[4]

Daily Dosage

Vitamin C	1,000 mg
Vitamin E	400 IU
Ginkgo biloba	100 to 200 mg
Selenium	30× potency. Drop 4 to 5 pellets into the container's cap, then drop them under the tongue and suck until they dissolve (they must not be touched with the hand). Repeat twice daily for 1 week. Stop if no results are obtained in that time. If you would rather not use a homeopathic remedy, or don't have access to it, use a conventional 200-mcg selenium mineral supplement.

Notes

1. Watson, Cynthia Mervis. (1993). *Love Potions* (p. 112). Los Angeles: Jeremy P. Tarcher.
2. Cheraskin, E., et al. (1976). Daily vitamin C consumption and fatigability. *Journal of the American Geriatric Society* 24(3), 136–137. Cited in Werbach, Melvyn R. (1993). *Nutritional Influences on Illness*, 2nd Edition (p. 285). Tarzana, CA: Third Line Press.
3. Sikora, R., et al. (1989). Ginkgo biloba extract in the treatment of erectile dysfunction. *Journal of Urology* 141, 188A. Cited in Murray, Frank. (1993). *Ginkgo Biloba*. New Canaan, CT: Keats.
4. Watson, p. 179.

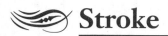 # Stroke

The medical name for stroke is cardiovascular accident. The accident is either a clot that blocks a blood vessel in the brain, cutting off blood flow and therefore oxygen and nutrients to brain tissue beyond the clot, or a section of a blood vessel that bursts, spilling blood onto the brain and, again, reducing proper blood flow to the area beyond the break.

Depending on what brain tissue is affected, the results of a stroke may be loss of speech, loss of intentional movement on one or both sides of the body, or death.

No matter how long a person has smoked, and no matter how many cigarettes, the risk of stroke rapidly declines once a smoker stops smoking. In contrast, the risk of stroke among current smokers is more than twice that of nonsmokers.[1]

Another risk factor is lack of exercise: Vigorous exercise, even a recent history of vigorous exercise, helps protect men and women against stroke. A lifetime commitment of from 30 minutes to an hour, two to three times a week, is recommended.

Beyond throwing away the cigarettes and throwing on the tennis shoes, chowing down on carrots and spinach seems to be a trusty way to keep stroke at bay. When researchers evaluated the diets of 87,000 nurses, they found those eating five or more servings of carrots each week had a 68 percent lower risk of stroke than those nurses who ate one or less servings per month. And, those women eating spinach each day (isn't it amazing they found some?) had a 43 percent lower risk of stroke than women who didn't eat spinach as often.[2] Was it the vegetables themselves or the beta-carotene with which these two vegetables are richly endowed? The researchers couldn't say and wouldn't recommend taking nutritional supplements until more research proved it necessary. However, a major European research protocol called The Basel Study followed up almost 3,000 participants 12 years later and found cerebrovascular disease associated with low carotene levels in the presence of low vitamin C concentrations.[3]

And don't forget vitamin E for preventing strokes. A Japanese study which gave one group of subjects dl-alpha-tocopherol for 3 years resulted in 5.9 percent of the vitamin-treated patients suffering a stroke, compared to 8.2 percent of the controls.[4]

Thus, it appears that all three antioxidants, vitamins C and E and beta-carotene, are needed. They are most appropriately obtained by increasing your consumption of fresh fruits, vegetables, and whole grains.

One additional aid in stroke prevention is the herb ginkgo biloba, which increases blood circulation to the brain. When 112 geriatric patients took 120 mg of ginkgo extract daily, their symptoms of insufficient blood flow to the brain decreased significantly. Such symptoms included dizziness, tinnitus, memory loss, depression, and headache.[5]

Daily Dosage

Vitamin A	Increase consumption of cold-water fish, like salmon and mackerel, 1 tablespoon cod liver oil, or 10,000 IU of supplemental vitamin A
Vitamin C	1 to 3 grams or to bowel tolerance
Vitamin E	400 IU
Ginkgo biloba	120 to 180 mg

Notes

1. Kawachi, Ichiro, et al. (1993). Smoking cessation and decreased risk of stroke in women. *Journal of the American Medical Association* 269(2), 232–236.

2. Anonymous. (1993). Carrots, spinach and diet tied to lower stroke risk. *Medical Tribune* March 11, 3. Cited in Hamilton, Kirk. (1993). *Clinical Pearls* (p. 276). Sacramento, CA: ITServices.

3. Eichholzer, Monika, et al. (1992). Inverse correlation between essential antioxidants in plasma and subsequent risk to develop cancer, ischemic heart disease and stroke, respectively: 12-year follow-up of the Prospective Basel Study. *Exs* 62, 398–410.

4. Hata, Yoshiya, et al. (1993) Secondary prevention of cerebrovascular disease with dl-alpha-tocopherol nicotinate. Vitamin E: *Its Usefulness in Health and Diseases* (Mino, M., et al. , eds.) (p. 283–289). Farmington, CT: S. Karger.

5. Vorberg, G. (1985). Ginkgo-biloba extract (GBE): A long-term study of chronic cerebral insufficiency in geriatric patients. *Clinical Trials Journal* 22, 149–157. Cited in Werbach, Melvyn R. (1987). *Nutritional Influences on Illness* (p. 133). Tarzana, CA: Third Line Press.

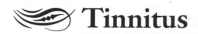 Tinnitus

There are many causes of tinnitus (ringing in the ears). One is interference with the microcirculation of the ear. The ear is among the most well-endowed organs in terms of blood supply. It is also particularly sensitive to a deficiency of oxygen, so anything that impedes blood flow can affect hearing.

A three-month study using ginkgo biloba extract for tinnitus and hearing impairments of various kinds resulted in from "good" to "very good" response in 82 percent of 28 subjects. In 53 percent of the subjects, the tinnitus completely disappeared.[1]

Vitamin A is also useful for treating tinnitus because the cochlea (the organ of hearing that looks like a snail shell) has a high concentration of vitamin A. The ear's sensory receptor cells are all dependent on adequate levels of the vitamin.[2]

Daily Dosage

Vitamin A	10,000 IU
Ginkgo biloba	180 to 300 mg

Notes

1. DeFeudis, F. V. (1991). *Ginkgo Biloba Extract* (EGb 761): *Pharmacological Activities and Clinical Applications* (pp. 11 ff.). Paris: Elsevier. Cited in Murray, Frank. (1993). *Ginkgo Biloba* (p. 27). New Canaan, CT: Keats.
2. Chole, Q. (1978). Vitamin A in the cochlea. *Archives of Otorhinolaryngology* 124, 379–382.

Varicose Veins and Hemorrhoids

Blood flows through the arteries toward the limbs in rhythm to the pumping action of the heart. Blood returns to the heart from the limbs through the veins, pushed along only by the movement of muscles and the general momentum of arterial blood pressure. Inside the veins are valves that keep the blood from flowing backward. These valves are fragile structures that can be damaged if you stand for long periods of time, if you strain while lifting or defecating, or if you suffer from deficiencies of nutrients that keep the vein walls strong and the muscles around those walls toned.

When a vein dilates (opens more than usual) and the valves are damaged, the blood pools in the area, causing an unsightly bluish, twisted road map pattern just beneath the skin. If these varicose veins are deep within the legs, they can be dangerous if they lead to closure of the circulatory system.

Hemorrhoids are simply varicose veins in the rectum. Hemorrhoids can be hidden or protrude from the anus.

Treatment of varicose veins in the legs and hemorrhoids involves moving more to avoid standing in one place, consuming high fiber foods that prevent constipation, strengthening the muscles around the veins to ensure the sides of the valves remain in proper relation to the sides of the vein, and improving the nutritional status of the veins themselves.

Dark colored berries, particularly bilberries, contain bioflavonoids and anthocyanidins (see Part I, "Bilberry") that help strengthen vein walls.[1] Supplemental bioflavonoids are also useful because they strengthen the walls of the blood vessels and help keep them toned. Vitamin C works synergistically with bioflavonoids, helping them do their job even better than they can alone. Vitamin E maintains the integrity of the vein wall.

Daily Dosage

Vitamin C	500 to 3,000 mg (if diarrhea develops, cut the dose by 250 mg per day until the bowels are comfortable)
Vitamin E	200 to 600 IU
Bilberry	300 mg
Bioflavonoids	100 mg to 1,000 mg, depending on the severity of the condition

Note

1. Murray, Michael, and Pizzorno, Joseph. (1991). Varicose Veins. In *Encyclopedia of Natural Medicine* (p. 539). Rocklin, CA: Prima.

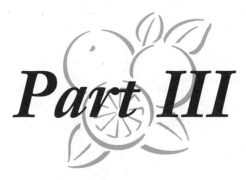

Part III

Gathering
Further Information

The old days of silence are over. Today, patients willingly express a desire to be informed. You want to participate in the decisions that affect your life, and know ahead of time what to expect from any one treatment, whether that treatment is a nutritional supplement, a pharmaceutical prescription, or a surgical operation. You also want to know the alternatives available. In Part III you will find some useful sources of information on treatment alternatives.

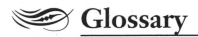 # Glossary

Angina pectoris Severe pain in the heart, often radiating to the left shoulder.

Antioxidant A substance that stops oxidation.

Arteriosclerosis Hardened arteries.

Atheroma A fatty deposit in a blood vessel wall.

Atherosclerosis A fatty deposit that blocks the passage of blood through the blood vessel.

Bowel tolerance That dosage of vitamin C just under the dosage that causes loose stools. Bowel tolerance dose is found by increasing vitamin C doses until loose stools results, then cutting back some each day until the bowels are no longer affected. The dose changes according to the health of the body. The greater the infection, the greater the bowel tolerance dosage.

Cerebrovascular accident A stroke.

Coronary occlusion Blockage of an artery exiting the heart.

Coronary thrombosis Blood clot in an artery exiting the heart.

Enzyme A protein that causes a biochemical reaction to take place, usually shortening the time it takes for the reaction to occur. An –ase at the end of a chemical name indicates an enzyme. Some of the common antioxidant enzymes are superoxide dismutase, glutathione peroxidase, and catalase.

Free radical A compound with an unpaired electron that seeks a mate for that electron by stealing one from other stable compounds. This process is what turns oil rancid, including the oil inside individual cells of the human body, and initiates many degenerative diseases and conditions, including heart disease, cancer, cataracts, arthritis, and aging.

Free radical chain As each free radical steals an electron from a molecule nearby, a domino effect occurs that becomes a cascade of thefts and the initiation of massive chain reactions that lead to tissue destruction.

Free radical scavenger A substance that neutralizes free radicals.

Lipid Fat or oil.

Lipid peroxidation Oxidation of fat.

Occlusion Blockage.

Oxidant A substance that causes oxidation, often with a result that is detrimental to body health.

Oxidation The process by which certain kinds of altered oxygen molecules cause biochemical reactions. Rust on metal and the rancidity of oil are common examples of oxidation.

Oxidative burst White blood cells use fragments of oxygen called superoxide and hydrogen peroxide to attack and surround invading bacteria until the bacteria are destroyed. This is a way the body uses free radicals to our own advantage.

Resources

We are capable of infinite possibilities
and become limited only when we shut the door on new ones
or when we are not aware
that there are doors we haven't seen.

—Virginia Satir

Finding a Nutritionally
Trained Medical Professional

American Holistic Medical Association
4101 Lake Boone Trail, Suite 201
Raleigh, NC 27607
919/787-5146

Medical professionals, mostly physicians, belong to this trade group for self-education and emotional support among similarly open-minded colleagues.

Price-Pottenger Nutrition Foundation
5871 El Cajon Blvd.
San Diego, CA 92115
619/582-4168

A library and resource center for nutritionally minded medical professionals. They also sell books and tapes, and publish an informative newsletter.

American Association of Naturopathic Physicians
P.O. Box 20386
Seattle, WA 98112

Naturopathic physicians are trained to use nutrition, herbs, manipulation, homeopathy, acupuncture, and other modalities, excluding major surgery or prescription drugs. The majority of states do not license naturopaths and so you may find one legally licensed as a chiropractor or acupuncturist.

Finding Health Information

Grateful Med
MEDLARS(R) Management Section
National Library of Medicine
Bethesda, MD 20894
TEL 800/638-8480; M–F 8:30–12 midnight and Sat.
   8:30–5 pm ET
FAX 301/496-0822

This service allows you to access on-line information from the National Library of Medicine to research medical studies published during the past 4 years.

World Research Foundation
15300 Ventura Blvd., Suite 405
Sherman Oaks, CA 91403
TEL 818/907-5483
FAX 818/907-6044

A nonprofit health information resource that can provide you with a computer search of 500 databases world-wide of conventional medical journal articles on any topic of your interest; photocopies of chapters and articles describing nutritional and other alternative therapies from their on-site library of medical books dating back to the 1600s as well as bulging files of clippings; an open-door policy for browsers in their library in their headquarters in Sherman Oaks, a suburb of Los Angeles; yearly international conferences bringing leading pioneers in the fields of nutrition and other nonpharmaceutical healing modalities; and audio-cassettes and books available through their catalogue. The Foundation maintains branch offices in Sedona, Arizona, Stuttgart, Germany, and Hangzhou, China, with which they maintain on-going contact through FAX and phone.

CANHELP
Patrick McGrady, Jr.
3111 Paradise Bay Road
Port Ludlow, WA 98365
206/437-9384

McGrady, fluent in German, French, and Russian, investigates new cancer therapies and clinics, attends international medical conferences, keeps up on the literature, and is connected to computer databases to enable him to provide cancer patients with up-to-date information about the best choice of an oncologist, a general practitioner with specialized treatments, or a particular clinic with excellent results for their type and stage of disease

Index

garlic and, 66, 149
ginkgo biloba and, 149–150
information about, 138–139
nitric oxide and, 7
prevention of, 137–145
selenium and, 49, 146–147
tea and, 72, 147–148
vitamin C and, 145–146
vitamin E and, 40, 142–145
Heavy metal toxicity, 57, 170–171
Hemeralopia, 189–190
Hemochromatosis, 35
Hemorrhoids, 202–203
bilberries and, 62, 63–64
Hendler, Sheldon Saul, 82–83
Hepatitis
cancer and, 120
vitamin A absorption and, 17
Heterocyclic amines, 114
Hippocrates, 189
Histamine, 36
HIV infection, 172–176
N-acetylcysteine (NAC) and, 173
vitamin C and, 173
Hoffer, Abram, 83, 186–187
Hoffman-La Roche Inc., 18
Homocysteine, 150
Hot dogs, leukemia and, 28
Howe, Geoffrey R., 123
Humphrey, J. H., 177
Hydrogen peroxide, 9, 83
AIDS patients and, 172
cysteine and, 56
Hydroxyl radical, 83
melatonin and, 60
Hypogonadism, 180
Hypothyroidism, 14

I

Ibuprofen, 192
Immune system. *See also* AIDS; HIV
infection; Rheumatoid arthritis
beta-carotenes and, 18
dysfunctions of, 177–179
fenretinide and, 118
oxidants used by, 7–8
vitamin A and, 177
vitamin E and, 178
Impotence. *See* Sexual dysfunction
Infant formulas, 50–51
Infections, 178
Infertility, 180–181
Insomnia, 60

Intermittent claudication, 45, 182–183
International Units (IU), 21
Iron, 35
Isotretinoin, 19–20, 79
dysplasia and, 124
squamous cell cancer and, 129

J

Jacob, Robert A., 27
Japan, Shizuoka Prefecture, 114–115
Jaundice, 17
Jet lag, 60
Jewett, Michael, 122
*Journal of Allergy and Clinical
Immunology*, 36
Journal of Nutritional Biochemistry, 158

K

Keratin, 166
Keratoses, 13
Keshan's disease, 146–147
Kidney disease, 74
Kidney stones
tea and, 74
vitamin C and, 34–35
Kleijnen, Jos, 70, 149
Knipschild, Paul, 70, 149

L

Lactase, 85
Lambert, Lloyd, 94
The Lancet, 173
Larson, Joan Mathews, 97–98
Laxatives, mineral oil, 14, 17
L-cysteine, 91
and cataracts, 157
memory loss and, 186
LDL cholesterol, 140
coenzyme Q10 and, 53–54
garlic and, 66
vitamin E and, 144
Lead, 8
garlic and, 66
selenium and, 147
toxicity, 170–171
Let's Live magazine, 144
Leukemia, 125–126
vitamin A and, 126
Leukoplakia, 127
Levine, Mark, 30, 31
Lind, James, 26